DELIVERING THE FUTURE

DELIVERING THE FUTURE

Reflections of a Rotunda Master

SAM COULTER-SMITH

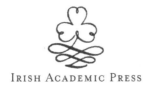

IRISH ACADEMIC PRESS

First published in 2022 by

Irish Academic Press

10 George's Street

Newbridge

Co. Kildare

Ireland

www.iap.ie

9781788551632 (Cloth)

9781788551649 (Ebook)

9781788551656 (PDF)

A CIP catalogue record for this book is available from the British Library.

Typeset in Adobe Garamond Pro 12/18 pt

Cover design: edit+ www.stuartcoughlan.com

Irish Academic Press is a member of Publishing Ireland.

I would like to dedicate this book to the amazing staff of the Rotunda Hospital who, for 277 years, have sought and continue to provide the best possible care to mothers and their babies.

CONTENTS

ABBREVIATIONS

AML	Active Management of Labour
CEO	Chief Executive Officer
CHI	Children's Health Ireland
CUMH	Cork University Maternity Hospital
GP	General Practitioner
HIQA	Health Information and Quality Authority
HSE	Health Service Executive
HARI	Human Assisted Reproduction Institute
HIE	Hypoxic–Ischemic Encephalopathy
IUD	Intrauterine Device
IVF	In Vitro Fertilisation
IRG	Independent Review Group
KPIs	Key Performance Indicators
MRCOG	Membership of the Royal College of Obstetricians and Gynaecologists
MSW	Medical Social Work
NWIHP	National Women and Infants Health Programme
NCH	New Children's Hospital
NCHD	Non-Consultant Hospital Doctor

NCHS	Non-Consultant Hospital Doctor
RAMI	Royal Academy of Medicine in Ireland
RCPI	Royal College of Physicians of Ireland
RCSI	Royal College of Surgeons of Ireland
SATU	Sexual Assault Treatment Unit
SHO	Senior House Officer
SIMF	Serious Incident Management Forum
SLA	Service Level Agreement
SpR	Specialist Registrars
TCD	Trinity College Dublin
TSCH	Temple Street Children's Hospital
UCD	University College Dublin
VBAC	Vaginal Birth after a Caesarean Section
VHF	Voluntary Healthcare Forum
VHI	Voluntary Health Insurance
VT	Vertical Transmission

FOREWORD

The Rotunda holds a special place in the affections of many people. These include tens of thousands of mothers who have given birth there; women who have been treated for gynaecological problems; infertile couples who have been helped to have babies; thousands of midwives, medical practitioners and other health professionals from around the world who have trained and developed their expertise within its walls; and health professionals all over the country who refer women for the specialist care offered by the hospital. Dubliners, too, take great pride in the hospital's architectural and artistic heritage, as well as its obstetrical achievements. The Rotunda, the oldest specialist maternity hospital in the world and one of the largest, is also one of the safest places on earth to give birth and to be born. This is quite some achievement for an institution founded in the mid-eighteenth century by Bartholomew Mosse, a man of singular vision and energy who devoted his life to improving the conditions in which poor and destitute women in Dublin gave birth.

Sam Coulter-Smith brings the story of the Rotunda to life and shows how the humanity and passion of Mosse are still inspiring his successors today. He recounts how as a student, a doctor in training, a consultant and master of the hospital he absorbed the values that make the hospital so special – the focus on the welfare of mothers and children; the collegiality and resilience of its staff, board and volunteers; the spirit of innovation; the willingness to adapt and change; the concern to improve quality; and the commitment to teaching and research. Of particular value is his account of the role of the master in providing clinical and executive leadership to the Rotunda, and that of his own experience as master from 2009 to 2016, during one of the most challenging periods of recent Irish history.

He draws attention to the many ways in which the special culture of the Rotunda, and other voluntary hospitals, is under attack. His mastership of the Rotunda coincided with Ireland's financial crisis and the resulting enormous pressure on public finances. While it is understandable that public bodies were concerned with controlling finances, the Health Service Executive's (HSE) unwillingness to assist the Rotunda mitigate the risks posed to the unprecedented numbers of women giving birth in inadequate facilities – some dating back to 1757 – in the hospital during those years is shocking. The manner in which the HSE managed the annual Service Arrangement – under which the hospital agrees to deliver specified services for the funding allocated by the HSE – is disturbing. The changes of policy as to which general hospital the Rotunda should co-locate with undermined confidence and point to a poor understanding of the needs of pregnant women. The establishment by the Department of Health of the hospital groups, without due regard to the legal and fiduciary responsibilities of voluntary hospitals such as the Rotunda, was another step in undermining the independence of such hospitals. Coulter-Smith also draws attention to the risks posed to patient care and to continuous quality improvement by the HSE's national electronic maternity record, which is not fit for purpose. The proposed integrated financial management system that the HSE wants voluntary hospitals to adopt is another step towards control, which will undermine the remaining autonomy and independent governance of the voluntary hospitals.

Sam Coulter-Smith's account of the challenges he faced as master of the Rotunda fits into a wider picture. The 2019 report of the Independent Review Group (IRG), chaired by Catherine Day, described the relationship of the voluntary sector and the HSE as 'fractured' and needing to be placed on a new footing. The group found that 'the pressures of the financial crisis seem to have led to "mission creep" and increased micromanagement by the HSE'.[1] In particular, the HSE seems to have used the annual service level agreement (SLA) negotiations to impose conditions that have eroded the autonomy of voluntary organisations. They found that 'almost all of the interaction between the HSE and voluntary organisations is spent on financial measures and targets, rather than on patient/service user needs and outcomes'.[2]

The report draws on the experience of other countries to show that Ireland is not unique in having a mix of different providers of health and social care services, and it highlights the way those countries have found solutions to the challenges of reconciling autonomy, service provision and accountability for public funds. The IRG considered that Ireland benefits from a strong public service commitment in both the statutory and the voluntary sectors, and proposed a new relationship between the two based on mutual recognition of their interdependence and shared values of public service. The IRG recommended a charter be agreed between the statutory and voluntary agencies to give official recognition to the legally separate status of the voluntary sector and to reflect its public service role in the provision of health and social care services. It also recommended that a forum be established to facilitate regular dialogue between the relevant state representatives and the voluntary sector to ensure their full involvement in future policy and strategic developments. On the vexed issue of funding, it advocated multi-annual budgeting, the simplification of service level arrangements, the resolution of the legacy deficits of some voluntary organisations and that the HSE should no longer be both a commissioner and provider of services.

While some progress has been made in implementing this agenda of reform, the outbreak of the Covid-19 pandemic in March 2020 required a singular focus throughout the health service on the protection of the most vulnerable. Although the crisis may have slowed the implementation of the IRG's recommendations, the pandemic has highlighted the strengths of the voluntary sector in responding to the pandemic. As Paul Reid, Chief Executive Officer (CEO) of the HSE, has acknowledged, and what a recent report by the National Economic & Social Council has confirmed, is that voluntary organisations responded rapidly thanks to their ability to take quick decisions, to innovate, to be flexible and to adapt swiftly as circumstances changed without the need for micro-management.[3] Sam Coulter-Smith's account explains why the Rotunda has the capacity to cope so well with the unprecedented challenges of Covid-19.

One can only hope that the wise recommendations of the IRG and the acknowledgement by the statutory sector of the strengths of voluntary organisations during the pandemic will translate into action to unlock the vice-like grip of the state over hospitals such as the Rotunda. The alternative – nationalisation of voluntary organisations or wholesale privatisation of the health and social care services – will come at a price, not least extinguishing the spirit that makes the Rotunda such an excellent hospital.

Ruth Barrington, PhD

PREFACE

When I completed my seven-year term as master of the Rotunda in 2016, I handed the mastership over to Fergal Malone, and returned to my former position as consultant obstetrician and gynaecologist. I knew to expect a big change for me, but to be honest I had no real understanding of what the impact of that change would be. The feeling of loss was like a bereavement, and not knowing how to fill the gap was a bigger issue than I had expected. I thought there would be a great sense of relief, but the feeling that one's *raison d'être* had been taken away was huge. I felt I still had something to contribute. I had learned a huge amount during my time as master and had gained experience from the job, but now I had no way of using that experience or those skills. And there was a lingering frustration that I could have done more. Peter McKenna, another former master of the Rotunda and one of my mentors, once said to me that his philosophy of life was that 'You are what you do.' At the time I thought this was a bit sad for someone who had achieved so much in his career, but I now understand what he meant. The importance of planning ahead for the next phase of your life is vital for all of us, no matter what we do.

I had planned to write a book about the history of the hospital with a focus on the past twenty-five years but was really not sure what it might look like or even how to go about it. When I started writing, I had no idea where I was going with the manuscript, so I just started at the beginning and recorded my own story. It was only as this unfolded that it became clear that there might be lessons to learn for others in similar positions. I can think of several situations where overnight your whole world can change – a politician who loses their seat at an election, a sportsman or woman who has a career-changing injury. In such situations there is a sudden life-changing loss of purpose and a void that needs to be filled. In addition, I felt I needed to get some things off my chest in order to gain closure, and I wanted to pass on my thoughts and my experience to others, and to illuminate to those who make the big decisions in government how it feels to be on the receiving end of their decisions.

This book incorporates my experiences of training in Ireland and the United Kingdom, of different health systems and how they affected me during my time as a consultant obstetrician and gynaecologist and as master. All of the opinions voiced are my own and do not represent the views of the Rotunda Hospital or the hospital's Board of Governors. No doubt others may have different views and may disagree with my take on issues and events, but this is my perspective on the last twenty-five years of the Rotunda's 277-year history.

It has been a huge privilege for me to have worked in the Rotunda and served as master. I have been blessed and so lucky to work with amazing colleagues, both midwifery and medical, in the Rotunda and the other hospitals with whom we work so closely. There have been ups and downs, triumphs and disasters, happy and sad days, but overall the quality of care and the services provided to women and their families has continued to improve. This is because of the people we have at the coalface, who achieve so much despite the outdated facilities in which we work. The Rotunda's voluntary status is what allows its staff to respond, to be agile and to adapt to the needs of our patients.

I hope this book goes some way to explaining how and why this sector of our health service is so important and must be cherished and maintained as our health service evolves post-Covid pandemic, post-cyber-attack and into whatever the next incarnation of health sector governance brings.

INTRODUCTION

My motivation for writing this book is to celebrate the Rotunda's 277-year leadership in Irish medicine and to highlight what we, as a voluntary hospital, have been able to add in terms of services for women and their families. I also want to explain what voluntary hospitals are, because their continued existence is being threatened by changes within the structure of the health service. I want to show how these hospitals add value and why they should be cherished and maintained as vital partners within our health service. My reflections and thoughts come from my experience as master of the world's oldest maternity hospital, from years of training in both Ireland and the United Kingdom, and from my time working as a consultant. My focus is on what we can learn from the past, what is valuable and what we can bring with us as we embark on a new journey post-Covid.

My seven-year mastership of the Rotunda Maternity Hospital, which commenced in 2009, was the busiest period in the history of the hospital, with more than 10,000 deliveries annually. At times the hospital was dangerously busy, with simultaneous emergencies stretching our resources too tightly. It was also a time of difficulty for maternity services throughout Ireland, with numerous reports on high-profile cases emerging and huge media interest in our speciality. The stress on the maternity service in general, and on the mastership position in particular, was very significant.

The country was going through a financial crash and public finances were stretched to the limit. We were working with a funding deficit and with staffing levels below acceptable norms due to headcount restrictions placed on us by the Health Services Executive (HSE). As a voluntary hospital, the Rotunda receives about 80 per cent of its budget from the government and the rest we are expected to raise ourselves. Government funding is administered by the HSE, which was established in January 2005. I went into the mastership with the naive idea that if I had major clinical risks or other big issues that needed to be addressed, I could go to the HSE, explain the situation and work with it on finding a solution. My predecessors had had direct access to senior officials in the Department of Health who helped them to manage challenging situations. I, on the other hand, had to work with the HSE and when I presented my clinical concerns and outlined the serious issues we were facing, I was told bluntly by one HSE official: 'It is your risk, you manage it.' It soon became clear to me that the HSE was not prepared to share responsibility for the unsafe situations that we were encountering on a daily basis.

It was only after I finished the mastership and the dust had settled that I began to reflect on the HSE's response and lack of support in more detail. What on earth did it think of us? Why were its officials not prepared to discuss our serious patient safety clinical issues? Was it because the Rotunda is an independent voluntary hospital rather than one of the state hospitals that they had inherited from the regional health boards? Money was clearly at the heart of it; the HSE officials would only talk to us about budget and headcounts, while we wanted to talk about clinical concerns, services to patients and resolving big clinical risk issues. Each year they would drip-feed us enough money to pay salaries and essentials, but we might not hear until late in the year what our funding for that year was going to be. This made it impossible for us to plan our way out of a growing crisis.

In 2019, a report commissioned by the minister for health, and led by Catherine Day, shed light on many of the issues that had bothered me concerning the relationship between the Rotunda and the HSE during my mastership. The *Report of the Independent Review Group established to examine the Role of Voluntary Organisations in Publicly Funded Health and Personal Social Services* (IRG report) acknowledged that there was 'a strained relationship between the voluntary sector and the state, represented by the HSE as the funding agency'.[1] Given that the voluntary sector was worth €4.7 billion in 2019, this is not good.[2]

Voluntary hospitals are locally governed, patient-focused, agile, adaptable and driven by indicators of quality outcomes for patients. They have their origins in eighteenth- and nineteenth-century Ireland, and were largely founded by charitable or religious bodies to provide medical care for the poor at a time when the government did not. Today these hospitals are still run as charities by voluntary boards, but they receive much of their funding from the government under annual SLAs. The hospitals also raise funds, which gives them independence and flexibility, but this independence is currently being threatened by an over-controlling HSE and, more recently, the new hospital groups.

Over the past fifty years or so, the smaller voluntary hospitals have been disappearing from the Irish landscape, mostly by being merged into much larger entities. While it is understandable that the state wants to generate efficiencies through these mergers, I believe that we are in danger of losing something valuable in the process. My professional life has revolved around the Rotunda, but in the very early stages of my career I worked in Jervis Street and the Meath, both long-standing voluntary hospitals which have since been relocated and merged into large teaching hospitals. For me there is something special about the ethos and the collegiate atmosphere of these hospitals. They have a character that is supportive, fresh and innovative. Indeed the IRG explored the special characteristics of voluntary organisations and found that they added value in terms of leadership, innovation, responsiveness, ability to make quick decisions and advocacy of service users.[3] While stating that the public and the voluntary hospitals share common values in delivering the highest standard of care to their patients, the report noted that the management structure in the voluntary sector encouraged a 'more prompt, flexible and responsive approach to problem-solving and supported the piloting of quality improvement initiatives'.[4] The governance in the HSE hospitals, on the other hand, is cumbersome; the IRG report stated:

> There is a widespread view that accountability and decision-making have become too concentrated at the top of the HSE. This can impede empowered decision-making and responsiveness at a local level in HSE hospitals and other services. There is often a very long span of governance and management control within certain HSE services. As a consequence, individuals in managerial roles have accountability without necessarily having the authority to make decisions.[5]

So, while voluntary hospitals are not necessarily better than HSE hospitals, nor are their staff any more or less committed than our colleagues in those hospitals, they have a governance structure that supports – and has always supported – innovation and new ideas to improve patient care and clinical outcomes. Their governance is close to the coalface, with a clear chain of command, is more patient-centred and not focused solely on financial control. This allows them to strive towards delivering better outcomes for patients. For this reason, the voluntary hospitals can undertake the sort of strategic thinking and strategic development that is lacking in HSE hospitals. Service planning is also much more effective at a local level.

For those voluntary hospitals, including the Rotunda, that have survived until now, government policies, such as the hospital groups and the major reform programme Sláintecare, as well as budgetary and micromanagement by state authorities, are steadily undermining their autonomy. No doubt there are officials within the HSE and the Department of Health who consider voluntary hospitals as different and difficult to manage, and would prefer that all hospitals operate on the same model. Of course, none of us is perfect, and we, as voluntary hospitals, have all had issues at some time or other, but we have been a constant in the ever-changing mix of Irish hospital care, and have initiated and delivered quality health services. A singular approach to hospital management by the state authorities does not serve the hospital network well as a whole, and the excessive control is having an increasingly negative impact on the day-to-day work of the voluntary hospitals. The IRG spotted this and referred to it as 'mission creep'.[6]

In this book, I not only celebrate the long history of the Rotunda but also state the case for voluntary hospitals, to show how vitally important they are to the Irish health service. These hospitals provide a quarter of all acute hospital services in Ireland and include the Mater Misericordiae University Hospital (commonly known as the Mater) and St Vincent's in Dublin, the Mercy University Hospital in Cork and St John's Hospital in Limerick. The three Dublin maternity hospitals, all voluntary, deliver close to 40 per cent of the mothers of Ireland, and other voluntary hospitals such as the Eye and Ear Hospital and the Cappagh National Orthopaedic Hospital provide specialist services. Pretty much everything good that has come out of the health service in Ireland over the last 300 years has come out of the voluntary health service.

The recent response of the voluntary health sector to the Covid pandemic may help to improve what the IRG called the 'fractured relationship' between the state authorities and the voluntary hospitals.[7] During the crisis, rapid decision-making was vital to manage the unprecedented and evolving situation, and the extensive network of voluntary health organisations throughout the country adapted with their usual speed and flexibility, showing great leadership and service throughout the pandemic. Paul Reid, director-general of the HSE, noted that the response of the voluntary hospital services to the Covid crisis 'knocked the socks off government ... that we responded in the manner that we did,' adding that voluntary hospitals 'can be a bit more agile for many reasons'.[8]

What we learned from the pandemic is that the hospitals and the people who are working on the front line did not have to be controlled. They did not have to be marshalled in any way by the HSE. All they needed was to be given the right equipment and the staffing levels and the facilities to do the job and they did it. Paul Reid agrees:

> I think we in the HSE got the biggest learning we ever got with Covid where there was a strong realisation that, okay, we need to give direction and oversight from the centre. But we need to let the services go at it ... and that was a huge lesson in how the system will just go and do things, a) with the right funding, b) if we can just unlock them, and c) get off the Powerpoint, get off the spread sheets. Covid has given us a big lesson.[9]

There are great people working in the health services who are well able to do a job. The Covid pandemic has shown that if you give people in difficult situations the freedom to provide the service, they will do it. The voluntaries have a template for how hospitals can work like this on an ongoing basis and work within a budget. However, to do this, the separate legal nature of the voluntary hospitals needs to be recognised and enshrined in law.[10]

The latest threat to our health service was the cyber-attack in May 2021, which caused massive disruption and highlighted the vulnerability of our IT systems to outside attack. The fact that in two consecutive years, 2017 and 2018, the issue of IT security was raised as a significant risk in two HSE internal audits is of serious concern. In the intervening period national IT networks were rolled out. These included the new electronic maternity patient chart used by four hospitals in Ireland. It appears that the goal to make maternity hospitals and units as electronic as possible was pursued without appropriate care and attention being given to the associated risks. Lessons need to be learned from this criminal incursion. It is interesting to note that, once again, voluntary hospitals were recognised as dealing with this issue much better and more efficiently than HSE hospitals, and were quicker to return to normality after the event. Part of this ability to recover faster is the ability to make decisions autonomously and to put in place solutions using their own staff.

If the voluntary hospitals were to be treated as a trusted partner of the health service, the impact on the Irish hospital system would be considerable. Formal recognition of our legal and cultural difference would allow us to continue to evolve and to spread our influence through the HSE hospitals. Already this is happening within the hospital groups, with the Rotunda, for example, delivering subspecialist services to the smaller maternity units in Cavan and Drogheda. But if voluntary hospitals are forced to take on the cumbersome decision-making processes of the HSE hospitals, they would lose the ability to respond and affect rapid changes in developing situations.

As I was submitting this manuscript to the publisher there was a significant development in regard to the future of Sláintecare. Two of the most important people involved in its planning and implementation, Professor Tom Keane and Laura Magahy, both resigned their positions. This has cast some doubt on the future of the programme. From the beginning, I believe that the proponents of Sláintecare did not fully understand or appreciate how important the voluntary hospital sector is to our health service. The pause created by these resignations is an opportunity to reflect on what we really want our hospital services to look like, and there needs to be an urgent conversation about how we create a health service where people are valued and where we can attract and retain the brightest and best of our trainees across both the nursing/midwifery and medical fields.

Today in Ireland we have a health service which is not bad, but at the same time it could be much better if the relationship between the state and the voluntary sector could be rebuilt 'on trust, partnership and on mutual recognition of need'.[11] Ideally the lesson we can learn from the pandemic is that the health service can be run on the basis of controlling what needs to be controlled centrally, while giving hospital managers a high degree of autonomy. As long as there are tight local government structures with appropriate accountability, let people lead from the front when it comes to the clinical side of things. As the dust settles on the Covid pandemic and the 2021 cyber-attack, and we look back to see what we can learn from these situations, I really hope that the value of hospitals having their own governance structures and a degree of autonomy will be apparent, understood and appreciated.

1

THE JOURNEY SO FAR

· · · · · · · · ·

The Rotunda is the oldest continuously operating maternity hospital in the world. It has been on its current site since 1757 and was one of many voluntary hospitals set up in Ireland in the eighteenth and nineteenth centuries to provide medical services to the poor, especially in the cities. Government health services were developed in Ireland in the nineteenth century but were usually dependent on the support of the local ratepayers and so the quality of the service was patchy. Meanwhile the voluntary hospitals pushed on, incorporating the latest developments in medical science and expanding their services through fundraising and determination. During the twentieth century, as government health services improved, the voluntary hospitals became part of the hospital network, providing services in exchange for funding. Yet they maintained their independence and their approach to medical excellence, with the focus always on innovation, the latest techniques and delivering the best patient care. As a result, they continued to attract the best medical staff and provide world-renowned teaching for doctors, nurses, midwives and other medical staff.

The Rotunda's history is still highly relevant in the twenty-first century, as it forms the background to our ethos, our governance and our drive to continuously develop our services. Since its foundation, the Rotunda Hospital has been managed by a master, who is a clinician with responsibility for every activity in the hospital and is accountable to a voluntary board. In the eighteenth century it was a straightforward matter to put all responsibility and accountability into one position because the hospital delivered only maternity services. Today the activities of the hospital encompass the full range of medical services required by women and their newborn babies – maternity and gynaecology, neonatal paediatrics and anaesthesia, assisted fertility, pregnancy prevention and termination, pharmacy, radiology, inpatient, outpatient, outreach, medical social welfare as well as the full range of laboratory specialist services. Despite the increased complexity and challenges for the master, the key to the success of this governance approach is still having one person in charge and everyone knowing who that person is. The master sets the tone for his or her seven-year term and makes sure that the board's strategic plan is implemented. Patient safety and clinical focus are paramount; issues and concerns can be dealt with quickly, with a lean management team overseen by a board that is clearly focussed on the well-being of patients. I believe that the mastership system continues to be a reason why the Rotunda works so well and I will look at this role in detail in Chapter 7.

***

Bartholomew Mosse, our founder and first master, was a man of clear vision and massive determination. The son of a clergyman, he was born in 1712, qualified as a surgeon in 1733 and worked in Dublin's new voluntary hospitals for five years. In 1738 he accompanied troops to Minorca during a conflict between Britain and Spain. On his way back to Ireland later that year, he travelled through Paris and may have visited Hôpital de la Charité, which had been founded in the early seventeenth century. On his return to Dublin, Mosse continued to practise medicine, specialising in midwifery.

Dublin at the time was crowded with people who had fled the countryside following a famine in the winter of 1739–40. Destitute, starving and diseased, they lived in appalling conditions in the city. In the course of his practice, Mosse encountered women giving birth in damp, cold and overcrowded slums. There were no public health services. Women gave birth helped, perhaps, by a handywoman, female family members and friends. Outcomes were appalling. In 1743, Mosse began fundraising to establish a lying-in training hospital to provide food, shelter and medical care for destitute mothers, and to train midwives and surgeons, with the hope of having a trained midwife in every county in Ireland. He purchased a former theatre in George's Lane off South Great George's Street and opened Dublin's first maternity hospital on 15 March 1745. Five days later, Judith Rochford delivered the first baby to be born there – a boy. During the twelve years that the hospital was located there, 3,975 women were delivered, 4,059 babies were born and maternal mortality was 1 in 90.[1]

Although he was working full-time in the hospital, Mosse was entirely reliant on charity and donations, so he had to put enormous efforts into fundraising, which included lotteries. He was remarkably successful in his endeavours and soon was in a position to buy a four-acre site on the newly fashionable north side of the city, in what was then Rutland Square and is now Parnell Square. Aware that private funding was critical to the long-term success of the hospital, the grounds of the new hospital were designed to host promenades, parties, dances and other social events popular at the time among the wealthy residents of Dublin – the income from these would support the hospital. The building was designed by Mosse's friend Richard Cassels, the renowned architect whose work included Carton House, Russborough House and Leinster House. At Mosse's suggestion, Cassels added the distinctive three-storey stone campanile with the copper dome.

The new hospital was opened by the lord lieutenant in 1757. The previous year Mosse had successfully applied for a Royal Charter on the grounds that the new lying-in hospital would become a national institution. This qualified it for government funding in a manner that would not have been possible had it remained a private charity. The charter provided for a board of governors, instituted the mastership system and established the Rotunda as an institution that could not, and still cannot be dissolved without an act of parliament.

Following the death of Mosse in 1759, the management structure he had designed fell into place and since then, with only three exceptions, the position of master has been held for seven years by a succession of obstetricians and gynaecologists.[2] The masters' contributions to the hospital are well documented and through these records we can trace the dynamic history of the hospital. Mosse's immediate successor was Fielding Ould, the author of what is believed to be the first textbook in English on midwifery, which was published in 1742. Ould completed Mosse's building plans, overseeing the construction of the round auditorium called 'The Rotundo', which gave the hospital its name, and the resplendent chapel located close to the wards. Both of these features supported the hospital's fundraising activities: the Rotundo by hosting concerts, recitals, promenades and other social events; the chapel by renting pews, delivering special sermons and holding collections during services.[3] The hospital remained a fashionable centre for social gatherings until the Act of Union in 1800, when the Irish parliament ceased to exist and the country's wealthy and influential citizens departed for London.

Meanwhile the work of the maternity hospital settled into a routine. From an account published in 1858, we know that pregnant women who wished to give birth in the hospital applied in advance for a ticket.[4] The women were mostly the wives of unskilled labourers, artisans, soldiers, seamen, weavers, combers, dyers, tradesmen, labourers and servants. A recommendation from a hospital governor, a clergyman or a respectable citizen was required. As soon as the ticket was issued, the woman was expected to attend the dispensary to have it counter-signed by the assistant on duty and to undergo a general health check. She carried the ticket with her until labour started and she needed to attend the hospital. A porter received her and noted her husband's name, occupation and religion and the ward to which she was to go. A bell was rung and a maid appeared to accompany her to the labour ward. When she was in the second stage of labour, she was brought to a low narrow bed by the fire where all patients were delivered. She was permitted to remain for one hour on this couch and, if there were no problems, she was carried to her bed which was made fresh for her reception. She was allowed to remain in the hospital for eight days. The only visitor permitted was her husband, and that was after three days. Often the women discharged themselves early. For many years, the Rotunda Ladies Committee hired cabs so the women would have protection from the weather on the way home; the committee also purchased linen and clothing for the poorest women. The larger wards, or Nightingale wards, are still in use today; these were designed for eight beds but sometimes ten or even twelve beds had to be put in each.

At first the infant mortality rate was high – from 1760 to 1773, 185 in 1000 babies died – but by 1800 the number had dropped to 35 in 1000. This drop continued into the nineteenth century, and by the 1830s, the mortality rate was on average 9 babies per 1,000 born.[5] At the time the new lying-in hospital opened in the Coombe in 1826, one in four Dublin births occurred in the Rotunda. The Coombe, on the south side of the Liffey, would help poor women in its immediate neighbourhood give birth in safer surroundings.

Of the numerous developments in the hospital in the nineteenth century, several are worth noting at this point. The first of these was Evory Kennedy's decision to create a gynaecology unit in 1835. That was a huge development and the start of changing the Rotunda from being solely a maternity hospital to being a women's health institution. Ultimately this brought us down the route that led to many of our twentieth- and twenty-first-century services for women, including surgical procedures on the uterus, ovaries, fibroids and cysts, as well as family planning, fertility, sterilisation and, most recently, termination. Maternity and gynaecology are two very different areas. From the early twenty-first century, clinical work in those areas has become more specialised. Now we have doctors whose main interest is obstetrics and foetal maternal medicine, some of whom do not do any gynaecology; we also have gynaecologists who do not do any obstetrics; and then we have a group of medical staff in the middle who do both.

The introduction of obstetric anaesthesia to the Rotunda in 1848 was another major step in the hospital's evolution. Following the advent of general anaesthesia in 1846, James Young Simpson, professor of obstetrics in Edinburgh, experimented with ether and in November 1847 began using chloroform on his maternity patients. Although successful,

14

it wasn't until 1857, when Queen Victoria requested chloroform during the birth of her youngest child, that it became more widely acceptable.[6] However the Rotunda adopted the new procedure early, and in 1848, several months after Simpson had used it in Edinburgh, the master, Robert Shekleton, gave chloroform to Eliza Hughes during the forceps delivery of her child.

As medical science developed over the following decades, the availability of a safe anaesthetic revolutionised other procedures, most notably the caesarean section; this procedure had been used since ancient times as a last resort to manage obstructed labour, but the patient usually died. In August 1889, Arthur Macan undertook a caesarean section in the Rotunda, the first to be reported on in Ireland.[7] At the 1890 meeting of the Royal Academy of Medicine in Ireland (RAMI), Macan said that he had read extensively about caesarean sections but had never actually seen one performed. The operation was successful and his patient was allowed to get out of her bed twenty days later.[8]

***

In the past, many maternal deaths in maternity hospitals were caused by puerperal fever, a pre- and post-delivery infection now known to be caused by the streptococcus bacterium. From the earliest days right up until the 1930s, successive masters struggled to control the disease in the Rotunda. Miasma was one of the suspected causes, and different approaches were used to tackle it. Joseph Clarke, assistant master from 1783 and master from 1786, introduced isolation and single rooms for women showing any signs of fever; at the time it was common for two women with their babies to share one bed. Clarke also upgraded the ventilation in the hospital and had holes bored in the doors and window frames to improve air circulation. Samuel Labatt, master from 1814 to 1821, had the walls whitewashed, the wards scrubbed frequently and introduced ward rotation. In the 1850s, gas lighting was installed in the wards, sanitation and hot baths were introduced, and a large, low-pressure steam sterilisation system was installed. Some years later, iron bedsteads replaced the wooden four-poster beds.[9]

In the mid-nineteenth century, Hungarian obstetrician, Ignaz Semmelweis, who worked in Vienna Hospital, linked puerperal fever to poor hand-washing practice.[10] In Vienna, as in Dublin, it was common for doctors and medical students to go from patient to patient, and from an autopsy to a pregnant woman without washing their hands thoroughly. William Smyly, later master of the Rotunda, joined the Rotunda as a student in 1870 and described the conditions in which the medical staff and students worked:

> In the wards there was a fire before which sat a group of students and nurses. Sheets were being dried on either side of the fire. There were no basins, soap or water. The expectant mother was fully clothed. For the medical examination she lay down on a bed and was covered with a blanket. The doctor dipped his fingers in a tub of lard and felt under the blanket. He then wiped his fingers in a towel and proceeded to examine the next patient.[11]

However, Semmelweis' theory about poor hygiene was rejected by many in the medical profession at the time, perhaps loath to believe that they might be the source of the infection that killed so many women. Of course, this was an era when information was disseminated slowly and often anecdotal evidence or a small study was all one had to suggest that there was something wrong or that there was a better way of doing things. Strong evidence was necessary to shift long-held beliefs and the information flow was simply not there.

It was Arthur Macan, master from 1882 to 1889, who introduced effective means to combat puerperal fever in the Rotunda. Macan had studied on the continent and had been a gynaecologist in Dublin before taking up the mastership.[12] Amongst other things, he taught new students how to wash their hands thoroughly with carbolic soap solution, blocked movement between autopsies and the wards, and kept a version of 'track and trace', where every person who examined a patient had to enter their name on a record so any subsequent infection could be traced. He also encouraged external palpation as a means of diagnosis instead of internal examinations.[13] In 1935 sulphonamide antibiotics became the first effective treatment for puerperal sepsis and, as they became available, the infection was brought largely under control in the Rotunda.[14]

One of the long-term outcomes of puerperal fever management in the Rotunda was the establishment of the domiciliary service, or 'the District' as it became known. On several occasions when the fever was present in the hospital, it was decided to attend women in their own homes rather than expose them to the danger. In 1876, Lombe Atthill formally established this service. He saw it as a useful way of freeing up space for gynaecology surgery, as well as an important teaching method. With the Board of Governors' support, he created the new position of clinical clerk, a post for young doctors who had completed their training in the hospital, but who did not yet have any of their professional qualifications; this post is equivalent to that of a senior house officer (SHO) today. The clinical clerk managed the records of the women being confined in their own homes and visited them daily during the week after delivery. The first clinical clerk was appointed in 1876 and that year 638 women were attended to in their own homes.[15]

The District continued until 1975; during the 1950s my parents met when they were both working with this service. By then the Rotunda District team included midwives and junior doctors, and they attended women in private homes who were within walking or cycling distance of the hospital. My mother, Joan Murphy, started nursing in the School of Nursing in Richmond Hospital. She qualified as a staff nurse and went on to do her midwifery in the Rotunda. She would have been a staff midwife by the 1950s. My father, Norman, was the clinical clerk. He had wanted to be an obstetrician, but the day before he was to go to London to sit for his Membership of the Royal College of Obstetricians and Gynaecologists (MRCOG) his father died, so he never fulfilled that desire. Instead, he went into general practice and worked on the District service to further his training. Although thoroughly supervised, the self-reliance and skills of the Rotunda District teams were well known. The District was considered a superb training ground for student midwives, medical students and social work students, and attracted medical students from Cork, Galway, London and Edinburgh.[16]

Healthy, experienced mothers were encouraged to give birth to their second, third, fourth or fifth child at home, but the women's own preference was also taken into account. Some women preferred to have their babies at home, others wanted to come to the hospital. In cases where there were medical reasons, overcrowded conditions, extreme poverty, lack of help or difficulty in coping, the women were actively encouraged to come to the hospital. My mother would go out by herself, usually on a bicycle, to a delivery, while a doctor and the Rotunda's district ambulance were on call.

There was minimal antenatal care in the 1950s and the District team had no record of issues and factors relating to the mother they were attending, so they never knew what they were going to encounter. The mother herself may have had no idea of how pregnant she was and, with no scans, she may have had no idea of how many babies she was carrying. My mother spoke of one occasion when she went to deliver a patient and helped to birth quads for a woman named Mrs Courage. That was an achievement in its own right – we do not deliver quads very often – but to do it in a non-hospital setting was remarkable. Years later one of my earliest multiple pregnancy deliveries here was also a Mrs Courage. She turned out to be related to the woman my mother had delivered on the District.

By 1975 when the District service ended, home deliveries were rare in Dublin. A series of new laws relating to the qualifications of midwives had been enacted from 1918 onwards in an attempt to phase out the use of unqualified handywomen at home births in Ireland. From 1924 it became an offence for a handywoman to attend childbirth other than under the direction of a doctor, unless she was a certified midwife. There were further acts of the Oireachtas, and from 1933 the doctor, a qualified midwife, or person in training to be a doctor or midwife were the only people permitted by law to attend a woman in childbirth.[17] By then, specialised nursing homes devoted to the care of maternity patients were becoming popular for those who did not want to have their babies at home and who had the means to pay for this service. The majority of women attending the Rotunda still came from the poorer parts of Dublin, where many families lived in tenements with poor hygiene, basic toilet facilities and very little heating. The Second World War, with its food shortages and difficulties in regard to light, warmth and transport, made hospital care more acceptable than in the past, and there was a considerable increase in admission to the Rotunda and other Dublin maternity hospitals. But also, by then, there was a much greater appreciation that hospital was the safest place to have a baby.[18] In 1957 there were 18,100 home births in Ireland, mostly in provincial areas where hospital beds were not readily available, and 43,142 births in hospitals and maternity homes. Ten years later there were only 4,139 domiciliary births as compared with 57,168 in hospitals and maternity homes. And by 1977 there were only 265 domiciliary births, most in emergency situations, with 68,627 in institutions.[19]

I was born at home in 1962 with assistance from Edwin Lillie, master from 1967 to 1973. When my mother went into labour, my parents rang him and he went to their house. My mother cooked for Eddie and my father, then went upstairs and laboured. When she thought she was ready, she banged on the floor with a walking stick and the two men came up and delivered me. All three would have had great experience with home delivery, but from my professional perspective, I would never have agreed to my mother having a home birth!

Although the District service ended in 1975, the Rotunda's external services continued in a different guise. As families moved from the city centre to the suburbs, the Rotunda set up community antenatal clinics. These clinics, which are still going, allow women to access antenatal care without having to trek into the hospitals; quite often the women have other children and transporting everyone to hospital would be a challenge. When I started in the Rotunda in 1987, an SHO and a midwife used to do the clinics, and I worked in Ballymun and Finglas. The women attending the clinics were in the low-risk category; the high-risk women continued to go to hospital clinics. Gradually midwives took over the management of the community clinics, and if there are issues, concerns or risk factors, the patient is referred to the hospital. In recent decades we have increased the number of antenatal clinics to widen the service to areas such as Swords and Darndale. This midwifery-led service operates five days a week from HSE facilities and continues to expand under Sláintecare (which I will discuss later in the book). A 2008 KPMG report into maternity services in Dublin is correct in recommending that we should be trying to provide a lot of the low-risk antenatal care in the community; it makes a lot of sense.[20]

***

The original Rotunda building has been extended several times since it was built, often when it was under immense pressure. In 1876 Lombe Atthill overhauled the layout and sanitary infrastructure within the hospital and was able to provide an extra thirty beds for gynaecology patients; this allowed an additional 100 women to be treated that year. William Smyly, master from 1890 to 1896, successfully raised funds for a new wing, which was opened in 1895 and named the Thomas Plunket Cairnes Wing after a particularly generous donor. Smyly, who was a fluent German speaker, had visited maternity centres in Britain and on the continent to gather information about the most up-to-date methods and equipment. The new building had two surgical theatres, one of which had a glass screen so students could watch procedures. It was also supplied with equipment that was novel for the time, including drums for the disposal of sterile dressings, the lid of which was opened by foot pedal. Smyly's successor, Richard Dancer Purefoy (1896–1901) had electricity installed in the new wing, which was extended to the entire hospital several years later.

Bethel Solomons initiated the next major round of building during his mastership from 1926 to 1933. Born in 1885, he had studied extensively on the continent, played international rugby for Ireland in 1908–10 while assistant master of the Rotunda, and was gynaecologist in several hospitals before taking up the post of master of the Rotunda.[21] His changes to the facilities in the hospital included a new operating suite and improved quarters for nurses. He created an X-ray department and reopened the Pathological Laboratory, which had originally been established by Dancer Purefoy in 1898 but had been closed since the end of the First World War. However, it was Solomons' success in persuading a reluctant Board of Governors to participate in the Irish Hospitals' Sweepstakes in 1933 that made the most difference. Through the Sweepstakes, the Rotunda received £160,000, which allowed Solomons to modernise the building with small rooms for private patients, a new nurses home, student facilities, a library, a post-mortem room, a mortuary, a lavatory block, sluice rooms, more bathrooms, an internal telephone system, new kitchens and electronically heated insulated trolleys, so that the patients could have hot meals. In 1933 Solomons also appointed Dr Brian Crichton as the first paediatrician to the Rotunda. A new ward for premature babies was added, containing an air humidifier and a small operating theatre.

In the 1950s and early 1960s, significant new services were developed, including paediatric, neonatal and outpatient services. The Rotunda Hospital was fortunate in owning the entire Parnell Square site and the Rotunda's architect, Alan Hope, designed several major structures for the hospital including the paediatric buildings on the north side of Parnell Square, the single-storey outpatient department along Parnell Square East, the new Master's House and the top-floor extension of the Plunket Cairnes Wing. When the original master's quarters were vacated, offices and wards for private patients were constructed in that space.

In 1967, Edwin Lillie drew up plans for a new five-storey extension, as a steadily increasing number of women were choosing to have their babies in a hospital with operating facilities rather than in one of the maternity nursing homes. Lillie's plans were never realised; instead, new outpatients' facilities were opened in 1985 and a three-storey extension was built in 1993. This provided an additional delivery suite, twin operating theatres and a new reception and admissions area. While negotiating for funds for these developments, Lillie arranged the replacement of the hospital roof, and, later, George Henry undertook an extensive renovation of the eighteenth-century Pillar Room to turn it into a conference and teaching centre. After that work had been completed, dry rot was unexpectedly discovered in the Pillar Room and further work was required during Michael Darling's mastership.

The Rotunda continues to own the Parnell Square site but, in preparation for the fiftieth anniversary of the 1916 Rising, the north-east portion of the site was given to the state for the Garden of Remembrance, which was opened in 1966.

Today, the facilities of the Rotunda are once again under immense pressure. With so many different services being delivered, the building is cramped and out of date, and the eighteenth-century Nightingale-style wards are still in use. Over the last twenty-five years, successive masters have been trying to get the Department of Health and the HSE to support the building of a new extension on the west side of the square. Progress on this has been delayed because of proposals around co-location of the maternity hospitals to acute hospital sites. It is clear now that any co-location of the Rotunda is many years away so development of the hospital is vital, as it will allow us to move much of our patient care out of the oldest part of the building. The eighteenth-century structure is no longer fit for purpose but cannot be extensively renovated as it is a protected building. A modern facility designed to cope with increased obstetric activity and a surge in demand for gynaecology services taking into account infection prevention and control standards is urgently required.

Our challenge is to get agreement from all the interested parties. As a hospital we want the best possible facilities for our patients and our staff. Dublin City Council planners have previously said they want any development to mirror the houses on the outer aspect of the square in terms of the height of the extension and stretching along the full length of the west side of Parnell Square. They also indicated they would like to see visual, if not actual, public access to the gardens in the centre of the square. The HSE and the Department of Health clearly have an eye on the budget and only want to spend what is required. Our task now is to manage all these expectations.

The 2008 KPMG report recommended that the Rotunda should co-locate with the Mater on Eccles Street, which is less than a kilometre away.[22] Then in 2015, arising out of the creation of hospital groups two years earlier, it was suggested that we should co-locate with the James Connolly Hospital in Blanchardstown. There are strong clinical links between the Rotunda and the Mater based on our geographical proximity and the large number of joint clinical appointments between the two hospitals. These links have been crucial to our success in managing patients with complex medical issues, and must be maintained and strengthened. Connolly Hospital cannot support us clinically in its current form. Staying in Parnell Square is a reality for us at this stage but making progress on developing the hospital has been frustratingly difficult as so many agendas have to align: Dublin City Council, the HSE, the HSE Estates, the Department of Health and the Department of Finance, and of course government policy has to prioritise maternity services. The creation of hospital groups has added further to the confusion by removing the Mater from the North East or RCSI Group, and I will talk more about this in Chapter 11.

All the while we continue to work from a very old hospital which, despite all the improvements we have made, still requires significant modernisation to bring it up to today's infection-control standards. The recent issues around the Covid-19 pandemic have emphasised how problematic and even dangerous it is to manage major infection-control concerns for mothers and babies in a facility that is too small for the purpose. Currently a plan is being negotiated with the HSE and the Department of Health for a modified west wing extension to deal with some of our clinical needs. With any co-location unlikely to happen quickly, the west wing development is vital to the delivery of safe and quality care to our mothers and babies. Our current master, Fergal Malone, continues to press the case and deserves great credit for advancing it further than any of his predecessors. It is not quite over the line yet but the need for it cannot be overemphasised.

2

CENTRE OF EXCELLENCE

●●●●●●●●●●

Teaching, training and improving standards of care have been at the heart of the Rotunda's work from the time it was created. Our number one priority is to look after women and babies, and it is vital that we prepare the next generation of professionals with the skills required to continue that legacy. The Rotunda Hospital is a teaching hospital with valuable links to the Royal College of Surgeons of Ireland (RCSI) and Trinity College Dublin (TCD). This role is central to the quality of the services that we provide.

I came to the Rotunda as a medical student in 1985. As a junior doctor I worked in two other voluntary hospitals and a statutory hospital before returning to the Rotunda as an SHO. I experienced first-hand the value of the voluntary hospital atmosphere, where the intangible ethos was one in which a young, ambitious doctor could flourish supported by consultants, midwives and nurses, and hospital management. The young doctors who joined around the same time as me were competitive and high achievers, all wanting to gain experience, deliver good outcomes and contribute positively to the profession. My experience in the statutory hospital in the second half of my internship was more difficult; it was bigger, less personal, more territorial and there was not the same level of collegiality.

Today the teaching role of the Rotunda is under threat from several sources, the most pressing of which is the increased demand for maternity services. This demand forces a reduction in the level of gynaecology services as the two compete for space, but if we lose or downgrade our gynaecology services, we will lose our status as a teaching hospital. Training up-and-coming junior doctors requires giving them exposure to the full range of gynaecology services. When our waiting lists become too long, patients suffer, and our teaching role and international status are threatened. This has happened several times in recent decades. During my mastership the board agreed to use discretionary funds to outsource gynaecological cases on our waiting lists to the Mater Private because of the increased demand for gynae services, which we could not meet on site. Recently we have built an additional operating theatre. And in 2021 we established a new gynaecology unit in the former Human Assisted Reproduction Institute (HARI) unit; this has gone a long way towards managing the waiting lists, providing better and more appropriate gynae care to our patients, and facilitating teaching and training. Managing high levels of demand needs the flexibility afforded by the voluntary hospital model; it also needs the trust and financial support of the government to allow gynaecology services to be maintained, even in a crisis situation.

***

Midwifery is at the core of what we do in the Rotunda. Bartholomew Mosse's vision for the Rotunda was that it should be a training establishment for medical and nursing personnel. He was influential in establishing formal midwifery training and education in Ireland at a time when there were no standards of practice, no oversight, no qualifications and no governance structure. Fielding Ould, the master who succeeded Mosse in 1759, published his 'Treatise on midwifery' in 1742, which helped to establish the field as a medical speciality worthy of scientific study.[1] Formal teaching was introduced to the Rotunda by William Collum, the third master. Joseph Clarke, the sixth master, created the first official registry of students. Two complete courses on the theory and practice of midwifery, and on the diseases of women and newborn children were delivered every year. Over the following seventy-two years, up to 1858, 2,875 male medical students and 656 female midwifery and nursing students attended the Rotunda for terms lasting six months. Even more had attended for a three-month period, but they are not recorded on the register. Most of the medical students were Irish, but there were also some from England, Scotland, America, Germany and Russia. They were a mixture of residential and non-residential, and they were rostered on duty so they could observe cases of interest or importance. Either the master or the assistant master was on duty at all times and conducted the instrumental deliveries. The medical students attended the wards where they gained practical knowledge of obstetrics and midwifery. Later in the century, William Smyly talked about how, when he was a student in 1870, he would bribe the hospital porter and the ward nurse for an opportunity to examine patients.[2]

By the 1920s the Rotunda had been the centre for midwifery training in Ireland for some decades when several new lying-in hospitals opened in Dublin. The Coombe opened in 1826; others opened in Arran Quay, Mercer's Street, Peter Street and South Great George's Street but did not last more than a few decades each. However, these hospitals competed aggressively for students and staff, and this threatened the Rotunda's income as it relied on student fees. Evory Kennedy's response was to advertise the opportunities offered to students who attended the Rotunda. These included the granting of a diploma in the Art of Midwifery, a certification that the Rotunda had been issuing from the earliest days of the hospital.[3] Other hospitals retaliated with their own advertisements. An unseemly row broke out. The Royal College of Physicians intervened and decreed that the Rotunda had no right to issue a diploma. From then on, the Rotunda Board of Governors was only entitled to certify students as having satisfactorily discharged their duties while attached to the hospital.[4]

Undeterred, the Rotunda embraced developments in medical science, making it an attractive place to study. In 1835 Kennedy opened the gynaecology unit; three years later he established the Dublin Obstetrical Society. Originally, the society was intended to provide students of the Rotunda with an opportunity to discuss issues under the direction of the master or another senior obstetrician. However, word of it soon got around and other practitioners started to attend. The meetings grew and were transferred to the new buildings of the Royal College of Physicians. Proceedings were published, thereby creating an additional source of information about the latest developments in obstetrics. In 1882 the society merged with other medical societies to form the Royal Academy of Medicine in Ireland (RAMI). The annual meetings of the maternity hospitals at RAMI were lively and important events during the twentieth century, and still provide opportunities for information sharing and networking, as well as being the forum at which the current three maternity hospitals in Dublin presented their annual reports for comment and assessment.

***

The training of women in midwifery was incorporated in the hospital charter in 1756 and records indicate that between 1787 and 1820, 40 per cent of the students were female midwives. At one point the hospital encouraged regional authorities to send women to the Rotunda for training in nursing and midwifery; in 1773 women from Wexford and Limerick attended and qualified.[5] However, the place of women in the hospital was lowly. They were poorly paid, the female live-in staff and students shared accommodation with the patients or with the maids, and they had no dining room or recreational space to themselves. Nevertheless, by the nineteenth century the Rotunda School of Midwifery was internationally recognised as a leader in the field.[6]

When he was appointed master in 1889, William Smyly focussed on the education of midwives to raise the level of their professionalism.[7] The women's living conditions were improved and they were given their own sleeping quarters and a dining hall. A qualified nurse, Sara E. Hampson, was appointed lady superintendent or matron. She had trained as a Nightingale nurse in St Thomas' Hospital in London and was the first qualified nurse to be appointed to this role. She found the standard of nursing in the Rotunda to be very poor and many of the nurses too elderly. Some resigned and others were pensioned off to be replaced by fully trained, qualified and uniformed nurses.

The quality and status of the nursing and midwife staff of the hospital continued to improve through the twentieth century. In his final clinical report for 1932–33, Bethel Solomons praised the midwives, attributing low stillbirth statistics to the labour ward sisters' vigilance: 'the skill with which these sisters acquire the art of fetal heart auscultation and are thus able to give warning of impending danger to the child has always seemed wonderful to me'. He also noted that good nursing had contributed to good results in the management of eclampsia.[8]

30

In 1939, when there were capital funds available from the Sweepstakes, a new nurses' home was built on site with ninety bedrooms, a pleasant recreation room and a lecture room. Student midwives received lectures from the master and his assistant, the sister tutor and ward sisters.

The increase in the standards of training and skills of midwives in Ireland was supported by legislation. In 1950 An Bord Altranais was established and became the regulator for midwifery and nursing. In the Rotunda the midwives went from strength to strength, monitoring blood transfusions in wards, undertaking blood tests in the antenatal clinics for Rhesus group and blood type, and working with Dublin Corporation to roll out the BCG vaccination.[9] In 1960 physiotherapists collaborated with midwives to initiate prenatal classes for public patients to ease the fear of childbirth and teach postnatal rehabilitation exercises.

As the Rotunda School of Midwifery evolved, the majority of student midwives were registered general nurses. Their training was initially for a year, and they attended lectures as well as doing practical training. In 1983 the training increased to two years and qualified the midwives to work anywhere in the European Union. Around this time obstetric modules were introduced as part of general nurse training and the Rotunda offered a three-week module which meant that there was a constant rotation of general nurse students attending training in the hospital. Meanwhile, hospital midwives were encouraged to attend conferences and courses, and to become familiar with different departments around the hospital.

By the mid-twentieth century the Rotunda also delivered teaching in medical social work. The medical social work (MSW) department had been established in 1936 to help patients, many of whom had multiple pregnancies and lived in slum conditions. Undergraduate and postgraduate social studies students did fieldwork placements in the hospital and the Rotunda medical social workers gave lectures. In 1965 the Rotunda MSW department even introduced tutorials for final year clerical students for Holy Cross College, Clonliffe.

***

Practical training for medical students was well established in the Rotunda by the early twentieth century. As already mentioned, the hospital had close connections with TCD and with the RCSI, which had held its first general meeting in the Rotunda in 1784. From the early days, clinical staff at the hospital gave lectures, attended autopsies and collaborated on research with their colleagues in the universities. A formal link with TCD was established in 1865, when the university instituted the King's Professorship of Midwifery.[10] In 1945 TCD created a new appointment, that of lecturer of gynaecology to its medical school. Ninian McIntire Falkiner, master from 1940 to 1947, became the first appointee to this position. The relationship grew with the appointment by TCD of a professorship in midwifery with a teaching unit within the Rotunda itself. Although TCD began to use St James's Hospital and the Coombe for practical instruction, the college continued to send undergraduate and postgraduate students in neonatology, gynaecology and obstetrics to the Rotunda until the early twenty-first century.[11]

Meanwhile, the Rotunda was building up an enviable reputation for the excellence of its specialist training programme in obstetric anaesthesia, which formed part of the requirements for the postgraduate training scheme inaugurated by the anaesthesia department of the RCSI in 1975. That same year, James Gardiner, our first consultant anaesthetist, was appointed to the Rotunda.[12] Until that point, junior doctors had given anaesthetics. Now anaesthesia became its own speciality and, once that happened, the role of junior obstetricians in giving anaesthetics disappeared.

***

My own Rotunda story started when, as an RCSI undergraduate, I spent a two-month placement there in 1985. In secondary school I knew I wanted to study medicine, but I also wanted to play rugby, and a gang of us who were in High School in Rathgar decided that we should win the Leinster Schools' Rugby Senior Cup, and we went as far as repeating sixth year in order to try to win. High School was not known as a strong rugby school, but we were a good team; in 1979 we had lost to Blackrock College in the semi-final of the cup, having beaten them earlier in the year, and that was why we were optimistic that we were in with a chance. Sadly, we lost in the first round to Belvedere College after extra time in the second replay. I worked on a building site for the rest of the year, coached rugby and went to the Pre-University Centre, which was then on Merrion Square, to increase my leaving certificate points.

I started as an undergraduate in the RCSI in 1981. At that stage I had not given much thought to which branch of medicine I would follow in the long term. As part of our education, RCSI students did placements in a children's hospital, a psychiatric hospital and a general hospital, as well as a maternity hospital. I got a placement in the Rotunda, where undergraduates did ward rounds and attended bedside teaching, lectures and tutorials within the hospital. We also attended some clinical meetings as part of our training, but only as observers, and got scrubbed up and went into operating theatres to watch what was going on. We had to do about ten deliveries and, in preparation for those, we had to observe five. I knew many of the midwives from having worked in the Rotunda gardens and as a hospital porter during my college summers, and they allowed me to do deliveries with them immediately. It was a great experience and I did more deliveries than most students would have done. For the first time as a student, I felt I was doing something useful rather than just standing back and watching.

When I graduated in 1987, I got an internship, my first proper job, in Jervis Street Hospital, a voluntary, general hospital and the oldest in Dublin. The hospital model in Dublin was different then: there were a lot of small, mainly voluntary hospitals in the city and they all took turns to be on call or 'On Take' for the north side of the city. 'On Take' occurred every tenth night and was horrendously busy. Over the course of the following week, the patients who had come in that night would be looked after, operated on, their medical issues sorted out and then they would be discharged. It was a very different model to the one we have now, where we have fewer hospitals, and these are always on call. There was probably more duplication within smaller hospitals and it may not have been as efficient in terms of managing investigations, but there were no trolley issues because there were enough beds within the system for the population.

During the year that I was there, Jervis Street and the Richmond, another old voluntary hospital, were merged and moved to become part of the new Beaumont Hospital. Beaumont is an example of a hybrid hospital; it retained the voluntary hospital concept of a board, but now that board was to be appointed by the minister for health. Jervis Street and Richmond hospitals lost their voluntary status and, eventually, their identity. In 1987–88, I spent the first half of my internship in Jervis Street and the second half in Beaumont. It was a difficult transition, with all sorts of teething problems and turf wars in merging departments. For example, radiology became a combined Richmond and Jervis Street department, with consultants and radiographers from both hospitals working there, and as a Jervis Street intern, I found I was at a disadvantage when looking for an X-ray from a Richmond radiologist.

I also found it difficult on a personal level. I had come from a small hospital where everybody knew each other, worked and communicated with each other, where we had our own canteen with terrific food, and our own nursing school, nursing students and medical students. Now I was in a much larger and more impersonal environment where it was more difficult to organise things. At the time I was too concerned with day-to-day matters to pay much attention to a bigger picture, but even then I knew that something good we had had in Jervis Street was slipping away.

On completing my internship in 1988, I still saw myself following my father's footsteps into general practice, and the idea was to get some training in lots of different areas. There were very few GP training-scheme places available at that time. I applied for one but did not get it. So, instead, I put together my own training plan, applying for jobs six months here and six months there. The first of these was as a casualty officer in the Meath Hospital on Heytesbury Street. My interview with Derek Robinson, the lead casualty consultant, was friendly and informal, at the end of which he asked me when I wanted to start. It was another small voluntary hospital with a family atmosphere. I thoroughly enjoyed my time there and even thought about doing Accident and Emergency as a career.

However, I continued to pursue my training for general practice and, knowing that I would need some experience working with babies, I successfully applied for a neonatal SHO position in the Rotunda in 1989.

That was the start of the journey. I fell in love with obstetrics and with the hospital. I was working with my hands and being useful, and I could see that no matter how far up the food chain one went, obstetricians kept working at a practical level. The neonatal unit was in an old part of the hospital and was being run by consultant neonatologists Professor Thomas (Tom) Matthews and Professor Thomas Clarke. Tom Matthews had been appointed to what was then a new unit in 1979 by the master, Ian Dalrymple. The Rotunda had employed paediatricians since 1927, but neonatology, although a recognised speciality, was still in its infancy. All spare funds in the hospital for a full year were invested in equipment for the neonatal intensive care unit and paediatric department. Tom was very good at fundraising and generating publicity. Within a year of his appointment, neonatal mortality began to decline. I still remember when the boundaries of viability were twenty-six to twenty-seven weeks. Now we are down to twenty-four weeks.

In the Rotunda as an SHO in 1989, all sorts of things came together for me. There was a relatively small number of staff, so it was easy to get to know people very well and they got to know me. The senior midwives, Sister Early, Mary Quinn, Sylvia Graham, Kate Creed and Fidelma O'Carroll, were very experienced and I learned a huge amount from them. There were some super staff midwives, who would still have been on the learning curve but were terrific colleagues, and we had great fun, both professionally and socially. The registrars were a very skilled group and included Chris Fitzpatrick, who went on to be master of the Coombe; Aidan Halligan, who went on to become deputy chief medical officer in England; Carole Barry Kinsella, a lecturer who went on to become a consultant in the Rotunda; Chris King, who became a consultant in Donegal; and Marie Milner, who went to Our Lady of Lourdes Hospital, Drogheda.

The senior registrars were Barry Gaughan and Mary Holohan, both of whom were later appointed as consultants in the Rotunda. Mary was the first female consultant obstetrician/gynaecologist to be appointed at the hospital. Barry knew me from Brookfield Tennis Club; he and I had been drawn together to play in men's doubles when I was about fifteen. He took me under his wing and gave me many opportunities, which accelerated my progress. Mary, too, was an incredibly generous colleague and teacher; she allowed me to do a lot in the labour ward while she did what I should have been doing in the emergency room and around the wards. All of this was hugely valuable experience. It was a very different time to today. We did not have to serve a long apprenticeship before we were allowed to take on clinical situations. The caesarean section rate was not as high, so there were more instrumental deliveries to do, and it was more of a see-one-do-one-teach-one culture. These days people have to see a lot more, observe a lot more and practise a lot more before they can get involved.

We worked long shifts. We were on call every fourth night and every fourth weekend, and always with the same people. We got to know what each one of us could and could not do. There was a bond from working together as a closely knit team, supporting each other through the good and the bad. There was also continuity of care for the patients, with accountability and responsibility in terms of their care. Those things are much harder to achieve now with shorter working hours and shorter shifts. When we were on call, we worked a twenty-four-hour shift, and then had to work the following day. I was Team A, which meant that I worked from Monday morning through to Tuesday evening every week. We also worked every fourth weekend, which meant that we came in on Friday morning and were on call until Monday morning. Therefore, every fourth weekend, I was on duty from Friday morning to Tuesday evening.

George Henry, who sadly died in 2021 as I was writing this book, had been master of the Rotunda when I was on my student placement in 1985. He was still there when I arrived in 1989, having chosen to return to his former role as a consultant rather than develop other interests or focus on academia. He was a great advocate for patients and everyone got the same care whether they were private or public. He understood the ethos of the hospital. He was a gregarious character, a great party animal, and famous for making speeches, singing songs and ensuring that everyone was included and involved. George encouraged us all to eat lunch together and he would often throw a problem out to the table. For example, he would tell us that he had just seen a woman upstairs with such and such a thing. 'I don't know what to do here,' he might say. 'Help me out, you are more up to speed on this.' I never knew whether he was not sure what to do and was genuinely pushing for information, or whether he was showing us it was okay to ask the question. It didn't matter – he was sharing and was not afraid of showing his vulnerability. For someone young and just coming through, it was refreshing. Obstetrics is one of those things about which you can never become arrogant, because if you do, it will come back and bite you very quickly. You are always a minute away from disaster at any time and that keeps you grounded. And George was one of those who rammed that message home. Besides everything else, that is probably where I got my understanding of how important the canteen is, how important it is to sit down, have lunch and share experiences, good and bad.

At the end of a tough day, we often went across the road to Conway's pub for a toasted sandwich and a pint (occasionally more than one). We also socialised together outside the hospital. We had a tennis team and a hockey team, and played inter-hospital matches. There were tennis courts in the Rotunda gardens and when I was on call with

Barry Gaughan at weekends, we would bring in the racquets and play; if the midwives needed us on the labour ward, they would lean out of the window and call us. There was a work-hard-play-hard atmosphere, which was supported by a warm, collegiate environment. My colleagues at SHO level were a fairly ambitious group, which generated a lot of competition. We were constantly pushing ourselves to learn how to do things, then how to do it better. The group included Sean Daly, who became master of the Coombe, Carmen Regan, a consultant in the Coombe, Hugh O'Connor, also a consultant in the Coombe, and T.G. Teoh from Singapore, who is now a consultant in St Mary's in London. I do not ever remember a situation where anyone at a senior level had to come down heavily on someone for not pulling their weight or for doing the wrong thing. There was a very strong culture of people being responsible and accountable for their own actions.

I remained in the Rotunda for two years as a junior obstetrician. Then I was encouraged to apply for a prestigious rotation that would take me to Hammersmith Hospital in London and on to King's College Hospital for their registrar training programme.

***

The path of doctors and midwives coming into the Rotunda has changed since the early 2000s. The number of junior doctors in training has increased, so the senior doctors do not get to know the trainees quite as well. Shifts and working hours are shorter. Consultants and other doctors are not on call quite as much as in the past, so young doctors do not get the same exposure to senior colleagues as I would have had. Nor do new recruits get the same level of clinical exposure we would have had at SHO and registrar level. The European working hours directive is responsible for much of this. As a young doctor, I would have worked up to 110 hours a week. Today, trainees are working 40–50 hours a week. We had time at the coalface and consequently developed experience and resilience. There was – and still is – an element of sink or swim when dealing with certain difficult situations.

Now young doctors are finishing their five years as specialist registrars (SpR) with less experience, less time on call and less exposure. The longest shift they would have worked would have been 12 or 13 hours, but when they become a consultant they are thrown in at the deep end and will be on call for an entire weekend during which they will be expected to practise solo. They have to have the physical ability and resilience to manage whatever comes up during those 48 hours. This can be stressful and difficult. The old argument is that resilience cannot be taught but has to be experienced. Every individual has to go through it and learn how to manage stressful volume situations, and how to go from a bad outcome to the next situation and give their best, even though they might still be reeling from the last one. That is harder for the younger doctors coming through because they would not have had the same opportunities to develop resilience and then they are faced with situations that put them under significant pressure.

In recent times there has been a shift away from gaining training and experience in British hospitals to taking up a fellowship in the American training system, where young doctors certainly learn resilience, but there are also problems associated with that approach. I will discuss these in Chapter 4.

In 2010, during my mastership, our long-standing affiliation with TCD medical training was severed when Professor of Obstetrics and Gynaecology Deirdre Murphy made the decision to terminate the undergraduate teaching link with the Rotunda and pull all of her medical students into the Coombe. As master I tried to convince TCD not to agree to the change, but I was unsuccessful. It was a real disappointment for me, and for the hospital in general, because the link was something we valued very much. But it was a unilateral decision and we could not prevent them from moving out. At the time TCD had students in the Coombe as well as the Rotunda, and it is probable that they wanted to centralise their teaching arrangement rather than have a wider hospital teaching base.

The RCSI took the opposite approach to TCD, in that they widened their teaching base and invested in teaching units outside Dublin, which in my view was a wiser option. Our relationship with the RCSI continues to be very strong. A clinical professorship with the RCSI goes with the job of master, and the college has a chair of obstetrics and gynaecology who is based in the Rotunda. We also have consultant senior lecturers and lecturers at registrar level.

The teaching of midwifery in the Rotunda is now associated with TCD, so the association with that university continues in the field of nursing. However, there has been a notable change in midwifery training over the past ten years or so. In 2011 the Nurses and Midwives Act recognised midwifery as a separate profession. It is now no longer necessary to do nursing to be a midwife, and prospective midwives undertake a Bachelor of Science degree in midwifery from TCD. This is a big change that has happened relatively quickly and, like any change, there are consequences. With our direct entry midwifery system, candidates come to the hospital with no nursing experience. While many are very good, very talented and ambitious, an element of their training is missing. Their teaching is all about normal midwifery, but healthy women become sick and unwell women become pregnant, and if a midwife has no experience of nursing, they may not recognise or be able to deal with these more complex problems. We still have some of the older experienced nurse midwives, but they are beginning to retire; now an increasing number of our midwives have no nursing training and this creates a challenge when it comes to recognising and looking after sick women. It is a risk for the future and I think we are poorer for it, but it was a decision led by the nursing hierarchy in Ireland. In my view this was unwise, as we need experienced nurses as midwives who can manage difficult and unpredictable situations. This is a decision that may, in the future, need reconsideration.

***

There is a reason why voluntary hospitals are the country's leading teaching and training centres. It goes back to innovation, best patient care and striving to improve at every level. In order to attract top-quality consultants and experienced nurses and midwives, the hospitals provide an environment to facilitate research and good clinical audit. Our ability to adapt, be flexible and agile, and respond to the needs of the population means that we can attract the best people to come and work in our hospitals. Sadly and unfortunately, although there are very good people working in HSE hospitals, they do not have the culture or freedom to evolve, adapt and respond with anything like the same degree of agility as those working in the voluntary hospitals.

3

IN PURSUIT OF QUALITY

● ● ● ● ● ● ● ● ●

Record keeping, reporting and auditing have been very much central to the work of the Rotunda since its foundation. Strong clinical auditing identifies trends and outcomes; it also identifies concerns over poor practice, unusual levels of intervention, unusual levels of complication, and also errors in practice. The concept of the clinical audit has its origins in obstetrics and the three Dublin maternity hospitals, the Rotunda, the Coombe and Holles Street, systematically use reports, data and scrutiny to plan services and for research. The Rotunda Hospital produces clinical audits every week, every month and every year to show exactly what we do and where we stand. Very few other services in the Irish health system do that. Good record keeping and clinical auditing contribute to our learning and to the way we develop our services; and we draw on our learning from adverse events to improve the quality of service we provide and to enhance the outcomes for our patients.

The levels of record keeping and clinical auditing practised by the Dublin maternity hospitals contribute significantly to the leadership role we play in Irish maternity services. Between us we deliver about 40 per cent of the mothers in Ireland each year, and the population growth in the north-eastern corridor from Dublin to Belfast suggests that these numbers will increase. This creates a huge amount of data. Historically, our maternity services have been copied for the way in which we do things. Of course, there have been blips along the road and we have great difficulty with funding, but overall we provide world-class outcomes and care for our patients, and our maternity and neonatal outcomes stand up to rigorous external scrutiny. There is no compulsion on us to publish our clinical results, but it is something we have always done voluntarily. Moreover, at an annual meeting of RAMI we present our annual clinical reports for public scrutiny by an external assessor and for comparison with other maternity hospitals.

The absence of strong clinical governance in any hospital leads to stagnation, poor planning and oversight and, in the worst situations, tragic outcomes, such as those seen in Our Lady of Lourdes Hospital in Drogheda in the 1990s, when a consultant performed far more than a normal number of caesarean hysterectomies. In a voluntary maternity hospital such as the Rotunda, high complication rates or particularly high rates of adverse outcomes would become apparent very quickly because of our rigorous reporting structures.

***

At a very early stage in our medical practice, doctors are taught that notes are a powerful communication tool and that we must clearly record a situation, the clinical findings and the plan for the patient. We understand accountability and we take on that responsibility as part of our job. When I joined the Rotunda as an SHO, I was expected to attend weekly and monthly meetings to justify and explain outcomes relating to my work. Midwives, obstetricians, gynaecologists, pathologists, paediatricians and anaesthetists were all present at the meetings, so there was a certain amount of pressure on a young doctor when speaking in such experienced company. These meetings continue today and create a culture in which everyone, from the most junior doctor to the master, is clear about what is going on. Time is allocated, attendance is expected, external benchmarks for comparison are available and reasons for less favourable outcomes are identified. The frequency of meetings ensures that any issues arising are discussed quickly. The data is fed into the annual clinical report of the hospital, which is assessed by an external expert and the findings are presented to a forum of peers from all three Dublin maternity hospitals for comment. This clinical reporting process also allows the master to keep on top of the many activities that are happening around the hospital, and allows the entire hospital staff to act with a unity of purpose.

The earliest Rotunda Hospital records were the ward books in which information about each patient and the outcome of their delivery was recorded. More extensive notes were made when there was a poor outcome, especially in the case of maternal deaths. In 1784 Henry Rock produced the first Registry of the Hospital.[1] In 1817 Joseph Clarke, twenty-four years after he retired from the mastership, published the first full medical report of the hospital, based on the notes and tables gathered during his period in office. In 1835 Robert Collins published a treatise on midwifery based on his observations during his period as master from 1826 to 1833.[2]

In 1880 the first annual Rotunda clinical report was published during the mastership of Lombe Atthill. The report is very much what we would expect today, with statistical analysis, case studies and references to major issues such as outbreaks of infectious disease. The earliest headline figures were the number of maternal and newborn deaths; morbidity rates were later added as a measure of activity. The annual reports became an important addition to the study of obstetrics in Ireland.

The modern approach to discussing our annual clinical report publicly began in 1882 when RAMI was established. RAMI was formed out of four medical societies – the Dublin Society of Surgeons, the Medical Society of the College of Physicians, the Pathological Society and the Dublin Obstetrical Society,[3] the last of these having been founded by Rotunda master Evory Kennedy in 1838. The Coombe, and later Holles Street Hospital, also presented their reports for scrutiny at these annual meetings, which were held in the Royal College of Physicians building on Kildare Street.

The same format for the meetings continued throughout the twentieth century. At the meeting, the masters of all three maternity hospitals stood up to defend their report, which contained a summary of the key events, key issues, key concerns and headline figures in terms of the activity of the hospital, including perinatal and maternal morbidity and mortality rates. The reports also contained chapters on the major morbidities associated with pregnancy and comprise an interesting history of medical progress and social commentary on what the relevant issues were. An independent assessor, usually from abroad, was in attendance and it was their job to highlight the differences, the good and the bad, and to open the debate. The master had to justify his position and take the flack. The audience could be very intimidating as it would include consultant colleagues, trainees from all round the country and former masters from other hospitals. This was a very important example of an independent external clinical audit and is a valuable national and international benchmarking system.

One of the advantages of the RAMI annual report meetings was that the three hospitals delivered roughly the same number of women and in high numbers. It must be remembered that these were – and still are – three of the busiest maternity hospitals in Europe. With high numbers, the analysis of that data produced significant findings. Big variations in outcomes were examined closely to ascertain what was happening differently to create those variations. The level of detail allowed us to assess ourselves against similar hospitals and find out what they were doing better so we could learn from them.

In the 1980s young doctors were encouraged to attend the annual meetings of RAMI. Although we were told that the meetings had become less contentious than they had been in the previous decades, they could still be quite vocal, with the odd bit of skin and hair flying. I attended my first meeting as an SHO in 1989, when caesarean section rates were still a major topic. That was in the days when there was very little movement between hospitals, so obstetricians and gynaecologists had a strong association with one hospital, and each hospital had its own culture. This created in effect three teams at the RAMI meetings and discussions became very steamy as each group debated the outcomes. Major arguments over caesarean section rates dominated the early meetings I attended, with Holles Street medical staff still very much against caesarean sections and concerned about the rising rates of sections in other hospitals.

The differences in neonatal outcomes also provoked some spirited discussion. In the late 1980s, Tom Matthews, who had supervised the opening of the new neonatology unit in the Rotunda in 1979, stood up and presented the neonatal morbidity and mortality rates and encephalopathy rates for the three Dublin maternity hospitals. Tom presented the data as relating to hospitals A, B and C, but everyone knew which was which. He became exercised about the differences in neonatal outcomes between the hospitals and highlighted the differing incidences of hypoxic-ischemic encephalopathy (HIE) between them. These differences were predominantly down to the way in which labour was managed and to the differing induction-of-labour policies. One hospital traditionally had a low induction rate and allowed pregnancies to proceed to at least forty-two weeks while awaiting spontaneous labour; as a result this hospital had a lower section rate than the other hospitals. Tom pointed out that the differences between the hospitals may have contributed to poor outcomes for some newborns in the long term. These meetings and robust discussions contribute to constant improvements in maternity care and to improved standards across the country.

Since 2010 or so, the major differences between the hospitals have all but disappeared, which is a good thing; now outcomes are broadly similar across the country and the RAMI meetings each November have become a little dull. Young doctors move from hospital to hospital to gain experience, so obstetricians are no longer associated with only one hospital. During Michael Geary's mastership in the early 2000s, all three hospitals decided to present their figures in a particular way with agreed definitions to make it easier for the assessor to extract information and make the comparisons.

Recently the annual RAMI meeting has become a full academic day to maximise attendance. The Junior Obstetrical and Gynaecology Society (JOGS) meeting is held in the morning, the Institute of Obstetricians and Gynaecologists' study day with formal lectures and presentations is in the afternoon, and the annual reports are read in the evening. It is an important social and academic occasion and an opportunity to catch up with former colleagues. In her report *Symphysiotomy in Ireland, 1944–1984*, Professor Oonagh Walsh stated that the RAMI meeting, 'is vital in shaping obstetric practice: it provided a forum not merely for discussion and placed Irish practice under external observation, but in the presentation of statistics and case studies of procedures, it provided an empirical base from which evaluation could take place and that is where its real value lay'.[4]

With staff from maternity units all over the country now attending, the event has been held outside Dublin. In 2019 it was held in Galway, but unfortunately clashed with another event that the master, Fergal Malone, had to attend. Lamentably, therefore, for the first time in over 135 years, the Rotunda could not present its annual report and there was no independent audit. In 2020 the RAMI meeting was postponed until December due to the Covid pandemic and was eventually held on Zoom. With tragic incidents attracting a lot of attention, the importance of these annual meetings cannot be overemphasised: they show that our clinical results are audited and reviewed independently, and this is why it was so important that the 2020 meeting went ahead despite the circumstances.

***

In recent times the dangers associated with the absence of records, or the lack of professional scrutiny of those records that did exist, were exposed during the inquiry led by Judge Maureen Harding Clark into the excessive number of caesarean hysterectomies carried out in Our Lady of Lourdes Hospital in Drogheda. During the twentieth century most maternity units in Ireland did not publish clinical reports, and even on those occasions when they did, questions arose as to where the reports went and who looked at them?[5] And if someone looked at them, did they understand the significance of what they were looking at? Could they assess the information accurately and benchmark it against other major hospitals? An uninformed person looking at maternity unit figures might see a caesarean hysterectomy rate of 2 per 1000. That does not seem like very many unless you know the rate should only have been 1 in 5000 when compared to national and international norms. Circumstances could explain an aberration, but anyone assessing the data needs to understand what they are looking at, what the norms are and whether there is an unusual trend in a particular hospital or unit. Our Lady of Lourdes Hospital maternity unit produced annual reports from 1952 to 1984, with statistics and other details, including the number of hysterectomies that were performed following caesarean sections. From 1984 to 1992, there was a small obstetrical section in the hospital's annual report recording the numbers of births, the caesarean section rate and gynaecological procedures. Then there were no annual reports until 2002.[6] It was during the period 1974 to 1998, but particularly 1993–95 when the unusual rates of caesarean hysterectomies should have prompted questions.

Dr Michael Neary joined Our Lady of Lourdes Hospital Drogheda in 1974 as a consultant. He was aged thirty-one, had his Member of the Royal College of Obstetrics and Gynaecology (MRCOG) qualification and had trained in prestigious training hospitals in Britain. But he had completed only seven years of postgraduate specialist training and Judge Clark wondered whether, in retrospect, it was enough time to develop mature judgement; she noted in her report that this level of training would be considered deficient today.[7] For much of the time in question there were three obstetricians in the Drogheda hospital, but it is clear from Judge Clark's report that they worked in isolation from each other. There was no designated lead obstetrician, no clinical manager and no one to review outcomes or ensure best clinical practice.[8] The monitoring of surgical practices was so inept that this bad and dangerous practice was allowed to continue.

Between the time of his appointment in 1974 and when his practices became the subject of discussion in 1998, Michael Neary performed 129 caesarean hysterectomies. In the Rotunda now we would do perhaps ten in a year, so most obstetricians would do one or two per year at the most. A comparison of the number of caesarean hysterectomies carried out in the Coombe and Holles Street compared with Our Lady of Lourdes Hospital in Drogheda between 1993 and 1998 was averaged at 1 in 4,373 births in the Coombe, 1 in 3,847 in Holles Street, and 1 in 179 births in Our Lady of Lourdes.[9] In 1997 Our Lady of Lourdes Hospital, previously run by the Medical Missionaries of Mary, was taken over by the North Eastern Health Board and several midwives who had trained elsewhere joined the staff. They questioned Neary's rate of caesarean hysterectomies, especially those involving young women with few children. The fallout was extensively reported on in the Irish media: steps were taken, Neary was suspended, then struck off the Irish Register of Medical Practitioners in 2003, and in 2004 Minister for Health Micheál Martin set up an official inquiry, which was led by Judge Clark.

The publication of the report in 2006 caused outrage and upset, although Judge Clark did have some sympathy for Neary. The report stated that questions about Neary's caesarean hysterectomy rate should have been asked in the hospital long before 1998; had there been systematic and regular clinical audits and reporting with appropriate oversight, and staff feeling that they could question unusual activity, then this level of intervention would have come to light earlier. Neary was practising in a unit where he did not get a whole lot of support. With better clinical governance, there would have been oversight to recognise that this situation was outside the curve. Had something like this happened in the Rotunda, the Coombe or Holles Street, it would have been identified very quickly through the clinical reporting process. No one would have had to work in those circumstances with those outcomes. Judge Clark's report repeatedly stressed the importance of regular clinical audits in her recommendations.

***

Our clinical records also play an important role in resource and service planning in the Rotunda. Making a case for additional resources to support increased demands or new essential services is based on raw data that indicates the need. This is relevant at every level, whether it is staff at the coalface who see a need to adapt a service, or the master approaching the state health authorities to get additional funding to support increased demands on services. Without raw data and an accompanying business case, nothing is going to change. This approach works very well within the Rotunda, with solid business cases leading to the establishment of new clinics and services, the purchase of new equipment, the appointment of new staff and other developments that are within budget and in the control of the master, the executive and the Board.

However, I found that it was quite a different matter when, as master, I tried to use our clinical data to make a case to the HSE for additional resources for the hospital. They were only interested in us staying within budget and headcount. In 2011, when we had the highest activity levels ever in the history of the hospital to date, I had all of the relevant data and reported the seriousness of the situation to senior people within the HSE. Clinical outcomes were not prioritised at our regular performance meetings and clearly the issues we highlighted were not being escalated as major risks to the upper echelons of the HSE. But even then I knew that, while information and clinical data was all very well, relationships were the key to getting things done. Maybe if I had been able to build a trusted partnership with someone in the HSE, the situation might have been different and our clinical data may have had some value in my discussions. However, during my seven years, I dealt with at least five different area managers. Consequently, there was no continuity, no trusted relationship, and no accountability on their part. After several years of trying to avert dangerous situations, I realised that I was not going to be able to develop such a relationship.

This approach has a fundamental impact on the quality of our national health system. Young, enthusiastic registrars and consultants who want to make changes in their hospitals can gather data, research their rates of interventions and their outcomes, and can benchmark against similar hospitals, which should give them an argument to go to the managers and funders and point out where their hospital is lagging behind. It is then down to the manager and funder to identify whether this is important. But even with an excellent case supported by solid data, the challenge to change anything is formidable. In the Rotunda, staff can approach the master formally or informally. Being so close to the coalface, the master is accessible. In turn, the master has ready access to the Board of Governors. Decisions can be made quickly. In HSE hospitals, however, the enthusiastic registrar or consultant will find it as difficult as we did to engage with decision makers. They will be going up against a well-oiled system that knows exactly how to keep them down, a system that will engage when it has to, then run them around in circles, and the medic will end up getting nowhere. There are so many good people working within the Irish health service who essentially become so browned off trying to change things that they end up resigning themselves to simply trying to do a good job; that or they go abroad. Sadly, it is only when a crisis happens that the state health authorities actually wake up and realise that maybe they need to do something about situations for which there had already been plenty of data to support a change before the crisis hit.

In 2016, arising out of the National Maternity Strategy 2016–2026, the HSE introduced a new monthly Irish Maternity Safety Statement, which was to be completed by all nineteen maternity hospitals or units in Ireland.[10] The safety statement gathers standardised raw data covering births, clinical activities, major obstetric events, modes of delivery and clinical incidents. While this is a good development, the outcome depends on why the data is being gathered and what is being done with it. Ideally the data should be available and analysed within maternity units so that each unit can use the information to examine their own practice and compare it with outcomes in other units to better their own service. But if the statistics are just going to someone within the HSE, the question then arises as to what the HSE is doing with the data and what actions will emerge from a review of that information.

In January 2017 the National Women and Infants Health Programme (NWIHP) was established to provide national oversight of services in maternity units, to identify areas with poor outcomes and to offer support to those units. In March Peter McKenna, master of the Rotunda from 1995 to 2001 was appointed clinical director.[11] Coming from the voluntary sector, Peter has a very good understanding of good clinical governance and put in place a system where all units in the country would produce statistics that could be compared and contrasted for benchmarking. However, there have been a number of difficult situations in women's health in Ireland since he took up the position, including the scandal concerning the cervical screening service, CervicalCheck, and much of his time has been spent dealing with concerns around these issues.

Nevertheless, with these recent developments it is now much harder for one maternity hospital or unit to stand out for being significantly different in either a positive or negative way. Since 2010 national clinical guidelines have been developed by the National Clinical Programme for Obstetrics and Gynaecology, with Michael (Mike) Turner, former master of the Coombe, as its first clinical lead.[12] Maternity units can audit themselves against these guidelines and identify significant service needs to ensure that we remain compliant. There is not much value in the new reporting system for the Rotunda, and it can be quite frustrating because it can mean duplicating information that we are already collecting and putting it into a different format, perhaps even with different definitions. However, as Turner noted: 'The guidelines were remarkably successful because in some cases they changed practices nationally. But what was really important was that hospitals which didn't have the resources to develop their own guidelines now have a programme that gives them guidelines they can apply.'[13]

***

Good record keeping is vital in all aspects of medicine and especially with regard to the patient's chart, which is used as a communication tool between professionals. It facilitates accurate recording of information to plan patient care and it is helpful for clinical review when required. In obstetrics it is vital, because collecting accurate information and the way it is recorded informs clinicians about progress in labour and can be used to predict problems often before they arise. From a clinical risk and audit point of view, therefore, accurate and timely recording of information is a key task for all clinical staff.

Medical charts and clinical notes in hospitals and maternity units around the country have evolved differently over many years and historically there was no standard approach. However, given the issues that have arisen and have been identified over time, it seemed logical to have a national approach to, and uniformity of, documentation. The conversation around standardising the maternity chart began early in the twenty-first century as reports into adverse neonatal outcomes were being published. A working group was put together by the HSE to move the idea forward, to take what was the best from each unit and to combine it into a new national chart. It was a good idea, but the end product was a huge tome not unlike an old-style telephone directory, which would have been too big and bulky for patients to carry, as well as being expensive to administer. Around this time the option of an electronic chart was also suggested. Many of us who had been involved in the process of standardising the maternity chart welcomed the opportunity to explore the idea of an electronic chart; we understood that all of the work we had done on designing the standardised chart would be used for this. The HSE set up a working group to move the idea forward.

The incentive and push for the electronic chart came initially from clinicians, who believed that, if done properly, the chart would have benefits in coordinating information from across the hospital and even, potentially, from hospital to hospital. An electronic medical record would also have advantages from an administrative staffing point of view. It takes a lot of people to manage charts, to retrieve them from the chart library, to track them, to make sure they are in the right place for the patient's next encounter, to file results and so on. The efficiencies that an electronic chart would bring in terms of reducing the levels of patient-services staff would be significant.

Unfortunately, however, the chart that finally emerged and its implementation process have created rather than solved problems. The Maternity and Newborn Clinical Management System (MN-CMS) digital chart was introduced in 2017. This has been, by some measure, the biggest change made to the way we work in recent times. As a profession, most of what we do is evidence-based; changes, when brought in, are usually monitored and audited before they are adopted permanently. Despite my concerns, and a number of people raising this issue with the national implementation group, there is not, nor has there ever been, any plan to audit or evaluate the safety or efficiency of the new MN-CMS chart. In my view this is a big mistake. Such a huge change in our practice deserves evaluation. Maybe it was not a good idea in the first place; a simple online search for evaluations of the impact of an electronic medical record suggests that there is a significant association with clinician burnout, as well as increased clinical risk for patients. But without any evaluation before, during or after its implementation, there was no opportunity either to identify problems or to explore ways of making this new system work to the benefit of clinicians, administrators or patients. The massive change was thrust on us and we, the clinicians, lost control of the process.

There are a couple of positive aspects to the new system. The drug prescribing section works well and improves some medication safety; and the laboratory results section is also good in reducing time spent following up clinical investigations. However, from an efficiency point of view, the simplest of tasks, such as logging on, requires multiple, time-wasting steps. We cannot use our swipe card to get into the system, which is standard Rotunda procedure to identify who is amending the chart, and the system does not automatically link to the printer or label machine beside the terminal, so we have to look around to find both. Searching the chart for information is challenging, as there are too many places to hide inputs, and every piece of data has equal value, so there is no clear hierarchy of the importance of a particular piece of information. One of my biggest concerns is that in the labour ward setting we have lost our old, well-designed partogram – the single sheet of paper on which a patient's progress in labour was recorded giving the clinician a picture for visual pattern recognition. It was an invaluable tool for recognising when labour was becoming abnormal and was also a great teaching tool for training doctors and midwives. There is a version of the partogram in the new chart, but it is poor and, therefore, not used well. The loss of this visual aid to clinicians and midwives is significant and adds to clinical risk rather than reducing it.

A further challenge for us is that the version of the chart that was purchased for the Irish maternity hospitals was a cheap, outdated version, and was not specifically designed for maternity services, so it is slow, clunky and contains hundreds of data fields we do not need. It is also hard to navigate and impossible to adapt because of its design. In addition, we as a hospital have lost control of the chart, in that we cannot adapt it or make changes to it for our own needs as all changes cost money and have to be agreed nationally. This loss of autonomy is a real problem for us as we have no means of adapting and improving the chart to make it safer and more usable. Handing over this control was an error on our part.

At this point the reader will have understood that I am not a fan of this particular electronic chart and I occasionally feel like a broken record when I am critical of it. As a communication tool, the chart is poor at best and when it comes to trying to understand the narrative of a patient's journey it can be almost impossible to get a clear picture of what has happened and how events unfolded. This raises major concerns for clinical risk, review and learning from adverse events, which historically we would have been so good at.

I have been openly critical of the chart and the way it has been brought in. My concerns have been batted away, usually with the comment that if people used it in the right way it would be fine. My answer to that is that the chart has to invite you to use it in the right way. It has to make life easier, not more difficult; information has to be easy to retrieve and risk factors easy to spot. In other words, it should make life easier, more efficient and safer but, to my knowledge, no evaluation or audit has shown any of these things. To date only four of the nineteen maternity units have adopted its use. Recently a decision was taken to roll out the chart to the gynaecology service in the Rotunda as well, again with no audit or evaluation of the impact of the chart. As a result, efficiency of clinics has been reduced, as it takes between two and three times longer to see each patient. This situation has not improved, despite us having used the chart for obstetrics for almost three years.

One of my main motivations in raising this issue here is not just to highlight my clinical and safety concerns, but also to highlight that this is a good example of how giving away our autonomy in even one small area can have huge implications. The cyber security attack in 2021 on the HSE and hospitals' information technology networks highlighted some of the weaknesses in the system. Our race to have the full electronic chart has brought us down a path where, because of poor planning and lack of investment in security, the risk of our system being hacked is significant. This was identified by several HSE internal audits prior to the 2021 cyber attack on the national health network but was not acted on. Lack of thought and the desire for the cheapest option has led to a poor product, which is not fit for purpose. And the lack of input from staff who work at the coalface has led to a system being introduced which is not patient centred, demands more face time with the screen, and forces clinicians away from direct contact with the patient.

4

PUSHING THE BOUNDARIES

· · · · · · · · ·

The voluntary hospitals plus Cork University Hospital and the statutory hospitals of Beaumont, St James's and Tallaght, are the seat of learning in Irish medicine. Virtually all guidelines, most academic research and information from clinical audits come out of these hospitals, and all national specialities are housed within these institutions. In Ireland a registrar or consultant with a focus on research is going to be drawn to work in a major academic hospital. They will want to work in a culture that promotes research and provides a level of freedom to pursue academic interests. If a maternity hospital wants to attract good trainees, if it wants top-class academic associations, if it wants to attract consultant staff, if it wants to promote midwifery research, then it has to have people and facilities in place to support the employees. And that becomes a self-perpetuating process.

Today all Irish maternity hospitals and units have broadly similar clinical outcomes so, in order to stand out as being the best, we have to identify other areas where we can do better and focus on those.

We can have good auditing and good research, and we can support everything necessary to add that element to the armamentarium of the hospital. With its discretionary income, the Rotunda has a culture that nurtures staff, provides training and development opportunities, and promotes research to find ways of improving our services and making things better for our patients. Our clinical data and research programmes are key factors in our success and, as one of the busier maternity hospitals in Europe, we have a large base from which researchers can produce clinical data. When our data is combined with that of the Coombe and Holles Street, both of which are almost as busy as the Rotunda, the Dublin maternity hospitals become a very valuable resource. Fergal Malone and colleagues from the other maternity units recognised this and created the Perinatal Ireland research group, which combines the output of all the major units in the country. Because of its size and the data available to it, the group contributes hugely to the international literature and has put Ireland back on the map as a serious player in maternity research. This is something to be celebrated, but, to date, it has not been given the recognition it deserves at the highest levels of government; this work should have led to our maternity services being cherished and supported instead of being starved of funding.

Creating the atmosphere and a supportive environment for research in the Rotunda is very important and the master as the lead clinician has to foster that involvement and facilitate people to do it. I spent some time doing research in London, but did not particularly enjoy it. Instead my strengths lie more in the area of clinical audit and clinical risk management. I saw myself as a master who would facilitate the research of others. Today the Rotunda provides a level of freedom to its staff to pursue academic interests that would not be available in HSE hospitals; staff involvement in this area is actively encouraged and their interests are supported.

***

Under the mastership system, the focus and drive of training and research in the hospital are strongly influenced by the master. In the past the academic focus of the Rotunda was on clinical outcomes and on practical clinical teaching.[1] The masters and clinicians sought out the latest thinking and scientific developments at home and abroad to improve outcomes for their patients. As innovative procedures emerged, the Rotunda responded quickly, introducing new clinical practices and creating new services. Many of our masters actively participated in international professional networks – in Britain, on the continent or in the United States – and several received prestigious honours from overseas obstetrics and gynaecology associations. Today ambitious young doctors would expect to spend time working in a major teaching hospital abroad. In my day it was usually an SpR post in a British hospital; now our direct links are mainly with the United States, where our senior registrars can pursue a subspecialist fellowship.

One of the outstanding Rotunda masters of the earlier period, Joseph Clarke (1758–1834), studied in Glasgow, graduated from the Medical School in the University of Edinburgh, attended lectures with the renowned obstetrician William Hunter in London, and arrived in the Rotunda in 1781 as a student of the master, Henry Rock. There he observed that the mortality rate of infants born alive in the hospital was considerably higher than in other hospitals; he put it down to poor ventilation, poor sanitation and women having to share beds. In 1783, while accompanying a private patient abroad, he visited London and continental hospitals to research these matters, and on his appointment that same year to the assistant master post in the Rotunda, he overhauled the ventilation and sanitation systems throughout the hospital. The results were remarkable; during his assistant mastership from 1783 to 1786, the mortality rate of babies born alive was halved.[2] He succeeded Henry Rock as master in 1786.

By the mid-nineteenth century, despite several outbreaks of puerperal fever, the clinical outcomes of the Rotunda had established a good reputation for the hospital abroad. In the winter of 1846-47, Ignaz Semmelweis, the Hungarian obstetrician who famously promoted hand washing to prevent the spread of infection, learned English specially to visit what he referred to as 'the great Lying-In Hospital of Dublin', but, unfortunately, he never made it to Ireland. In 1852 F.H. d'Arneth, a representative of the Viennese Lying-In Hospital, a leading continental school, visited Dublin and reported that although the number of deliveries in the Rotunda was not as great as in the maternity hospital in Vienna, it equalled or exceeded the numbers in the maternity hospitals of Paris and Prague. D'Arneth had visited the main maternity teaching centres and regarded the Rotunda School of Midwifery as the only one of real importance in Britain and Ireland. He compared maternal mortality figures for the twenty-year period of 1829–49 with Vienna at 5.35 per cent, Paris at 4.18 per cent, and the Rotunda at 1.34 per cent. He also noted that ventilation in the Rotunda was more efficient than in the Viennese hospital and that there were no foul odours. In 1854 the Danish government sent a Professor Dews to report on obstetrical teaching in the region; he also found the teaching in Dublin to be superior to the teaching in London.[3]

Many of the later masters had strong professional networks abroad through training, publications and association with learned obstetric and gynaecology societies and teaching centres. To name but a few, Lombe Atthill, master from 1875 to 1882, published *Clinical Lectures on the Diseases Peculiar to Women*, of which, ultimately, there were multiple English editions, two American editions, an edition in French and another in Spanish. Arthur Macan, master from 1882 to 1889, studied in various continental schools after graduating in Ireland and was a strong advocate of the Listerian antiseptic principles, which he introduced with good results to the Rotunda. William Smyly, the master from 1890 to 1896, who contributed significantly to the modernisation of the hospital, held offices in British obstetric and gynaecology societies, was an examiner with the Indian Medical Service, and was recognised for his work in Glasgow and Leipzig.

In the twentieth century, Bethel Solomons, master from 1926 to 1933, studied at Trinity College, obtained his Fellowship of the Royal College of Physicians in Ireland in 1914, and subsequently studied in Vienna, Berlin, Paris, Leipzig and other centres. In the 1930s he was recognised in the United States with honorary fellowships of distinguished associations.[4] In 1934 he was awarded the Honorary Fellowship of the American College of Surgeons and was made an honorary fellow or member of several other American associations. Ninian Falkiner, master from 1940 to 1947, was described as having an excellent record as a clinical researcher and being the author of 'arguably the best series of papers in reproductive medicine ever presented to the Obstetrical Section [of RAMI]'. Falkiner had also attended the British Medical Association meeting in Australia in 1935, and had visited centres in Canada, Melbourne, Sydney, Singapore and Bombay. In 1947, two years after it was scheduled, the Rotunda held a Bicentenary Congress; Falkiner edited the proceedings which 'remain a unique overview of obstetrics, neonatal paediatric and gynaecology as it related to sterility at that time', according to Alan Browne, master from 1960 to 1966.[5]

In the 1960s, following on from work undertaken in Berlin, amnioscopy and foetal blood sampling were researched in the Rotunda, with reports published on a large number of cases. However, Browne noted that a chronic shortage of funds for research and no staff members dedicated to this area meant that clinical research was not high on the agenda.[6] During his mastership, the main contributions to research came from neonatology and pathology. Although academic units – undergraduates from TCD and postgraduates from the RCSI – increased the potential for clinical research and publication, this aspect of the teaching hospital's activity was, according to Browne, disappointing, with the Rotunda's clinical reports still the main focus of the hospital's academic work.[7]

In 1967, the outlook improved when incoming master Edwin Lillie, supported by the medical staff, proposed setting up a charity fundraising arm. 'Friends of the Rotunda' was formed in 1971 and incorporated in 1974 as a body with a separate governance to raise funds for research, as well as for new equipment and patient facilities. A function formally announcing Friends of the Rotunda was attended by President Erskine Childers. Output of papers and projects increased, many funded by the Friends. In the 1990s these included cot death research, the study of congenital malformations, placenta studies, hypertension in pregnancy and the study of menopause. The Friends was renamed The Rotunda Foundation in 2016.

Brian Cleary, chief pharmacist, described one recent project:

This project, co-funded by the School of Pharmacy, Royal College of Surgeons in Ireland and The Rotunda Foundation, examined the impact of a neonatal research pharmacist on neonatal medication use processes. Through multidisciplinary collaboration with the NICU [Neonatal Intensive Care Unit] team, a medication safety bundle was developed that used multiple risk reduction strategies to improve the safety of the medication use process for high-risk neonatal infusions. The bundle, which incorporated electronic prescribing, standardised concentration infusions, smart infusion pumps and electronically generated labels with preparation instructions, led to a significant reduction in potential medication safety issues. This medication safety bundle has been incorporated into the digital chart, which now covers 40 per cent of Irish births.[8]

This is a very good example of how a keen, talented person with foresight can flourish in a voluntary hospital.

***

When I arrived in the Rotunda in 1988, the training available at the hospital had taken a step forward with the establishment of an international training rotation for postgraduate obstetricians and gynaecologists between the Rotunda and Hammersmith Hospital, a major teaching hospital in London. It had been set up by Michael (Mike) Darling, master from 1988 to 1994. He had spent four years (1978–81) at the Royal Postgraduate Medical School at Hammersmith where he trained under the renowned Robert Winston, a pioneer in the field of in vitro fertilisation (IVF). Mike worked on all aspects of the management of female infertility, particularly microsurgical techniques.

Mike returned to the Rotunda in 1981, was appointed to a consultant post in 1983 and appointed master in 1988. At that point there were no structured postgraduate training programmes in obstetrics and gynaecology in Ireland, no SpR posts and no formal rotations. Young doctors who wanted to specialise in a particular area were expected to patch together their own training by seeking out and applying for a succession of jobs. Mike recognised this lack and set up what may have been the first formal rotation in the field between Ireland and Britain for people in the early stages of their career. The intention was that once the postgraduate student was in Hammersmith, they would use it as a springboard to get into a registrar rotation in a major London teaching hospital where they would get full access to the British SpR structured training programme. A lot of people did that rotation and this was, without doubt, one of Mike's most important legacies to our profession.

I applied for the rotation in 1989. The competition was very tough, but I was successful and moved to London with my wife, Cathy, starting there in February 1990. It was a one-year appointment, with six months in the Rotunda followed by six months in Hammersmith. For me the appeal of Hammersmith was what it could deliver in terms of experience and training. Coming from the very general training available in Ireland, I was now going to get exposure to the subspecialist services of fertility, microsurgery and gynaecological oncology.

Starting as an unknown young doctor in Hammersmith Hospital on a six-month rotation, it was necessary to make a reputation for myself. At that level there was a balance between training and delivering the service, but no major decision-making, so it was just about proving myself through hard work. On a short rotation, working with fellow

SHOs and junior registrars, all at an early stage in their career, one of the most important aspects was the chance to gather experience and to learn different ways of doing things. Hammersmith had a relatively small maternity unit and did not do many deliveries. I would have been on call for obstetrics at night quite a lot, but it was not that busy so I was mostly doing gynaecology. As one of the major international centres for tubal infertility service, I was involved in the clinical and surgical management of patients and was learning tubal surgery techniques. Professor Sir Robert Winston and his colleague Raul Margara were my mentors and teachers. It was my first interaction with a major subspecialist service.

As the Hammersmith rotation was coming to an end, I applied for a three-year rotation at King's College Hospital, a large teaching hospital and at the time the absolute pinnacle of training hospitals in London. During the course of the interview for that post, I was asked if I would do a termination of pregnancy.[9] I was not expecting that question. My answer was that it was not something I would do from choice, but if it was deemed to be part of the work of the hospital and the department and it was something I had no choice about, then of course I would get involved. I was offered the position and started there in 1991. King's is situated in the south city centre, near Camberwell and Brixton, and there were a lot of unplanned pregnancies with almost as many terminations as there were deliveries. However, the surgical termination service was delivered in a day-care facility across the road from the hospital and I do not remember them ever coming to the obstetrics and gynaecology services. But it was a massive culture change to me. I was young, in a different place and it was exciting; I soaked up all of this new experience and learned from it.

Over the following three years, the King's rotation took me out to Kent and back into London. The purpose was to bring the doctor from one training hospital to another, and to district general hospitals, where we gained experience in looking after more normal-risk patients. There were still cases with complications in the district hospitals, but the very high-risk patients would usually have been transferred to one of the big teaching hospitals in London. None of these district hospitals were as busy as the Rotunda, but I was on call more often, so, while it was nothing special, it offered more experience, higher numbers of patients, more procedures, and further opportunities to work with different consultants, some of whom had special interests. There was a huge research department at King's hospital devoted to the area of foetal medicine. It was not something that I was particularly interested in because it involved sticking needles into pregnant tummies and doing procedures on babies in utero. On the other hand, there was quite a lot of gynaecology scanning, which interested me more, so I got involved with that.

By now I had completed the MRCOG, my final postgraduate professional qualification.[10] I was ready for a senior registrar role and was looking out for a suitable post in a good hospital. In 1994, when a two-and-a-half-year research post arose in the Royal Free Hospital in Hampstead to do gynaecology scanning, I applied for it and was successful. At the time there was a fertility treatment service in the Royal Free under Professor Allan Maclean and there was a suggestion that women who had had IVF or who had suffered infertility were at a higher risk of developing ovarian cancer. The research project was to set up a screening programme on a group of women who had received fertility treatment in the Royal Free and to see if there was a higher

70

incidence of ovarian cancer in that population. Unfortunately, medical politics got in the way and the project never happened.

Instead, I undertook a research programme into the prediction of malignancy in pelvic masses, which involved scanning pelvic masses, ovarian masses and ovarian tumours. I saw patients pre-operatively who had ovarian pathology and analysed scan information to see if we could predict what the nature of the ovarian mass was; during surgery we took tissue samples and did a range of immunohistochemical analysis, then correlated the scan data with the immunohistochemical data from the laboratory. The post in the Royal Free allowed me to do pure research, learn research methodology, develop more in-depth knowledge of a particular area and publish papers. Several years later, when back in the Rotunda, I started an ovarian screening clinic. What emerged over time was that ovarian screening is not particularly good at predicting the nature of an ovarian mass. It might pick up the diagnosis a little bit earlier, but it has not been shown to improve survival, so is not something that is pursued now.

On reflection, the British team training system in all the hospitals I worked in was still quite an old-fashioned model. They were big general hospitals and these were very traditional in terms of their hierarchy and training model. The consultant was king and there was a team working with the consultant – the senior registrar, the registrar and SHOs. The nice thing about those hospitals was that while they were busy, they were well staffed with all the specialties including gynae oncology, gynae urology and obstetrics, as well as more specialised work in terms of foetal medicine. I was meeting people who were at the cutting edge of research, writing the textbooks, giving the lectures and doing the teaching. Partly because the NHS was a very powerful and well-respected service, there were very few private obstetrics services in Britain, so the medical professionals were mostly working in the public service. The way they made their reputation was through research and publications and being regarded as the leader in their field, and they had the time to do this. It was nice to dip into that. In Dublin, in contrast, we were dealing with higher volumes of activity in our labour wards.

It was while I was in London that the European Union Working Time Directive was introduced in the UK and there was a move away from long shifts. That was the first experience I had had of shorter shifts and I hated them. I was used to working long hours and was quite happy doing that. I felt that shorter shifts compromised continuity of care and accountability, and it was not for the better in terms of patient care or training. I can see why people might argue that when you are tired you tend to make mistakes and bad things can happen, but my experience of the longer hours was more positive than that.

By 1996 Cathy and I were settled in London, but with two small children and our parents getting older, we had to make a decision as to where to pin our future. Cathy, who is a paediatric neuropsychologist, had a very good job in Guy's and St Thomas' Hospital and would happily have remained there. I was coming to the end of the research programme in the Royal Free and was thinking about whether my future was going to be in London, outside London, back in Dublin or elsewhere. Also, I had to decide what type of hospital I wanted to work in: a district general hospital where the work would be at the low-risk end of the speciality, or a teaching hospital with access to undergraduate and postgraduate teaching and training? One of the advantages of going away and working in other units is that it provides some insight into the choices one needs to make.

In fact, the choice for me was straightforward. I saw myself working in a teaching hospital of equivalent status to the Rotunda. A couple of opportunities in Britain arose but did not work out. During my time in Britain, I would always have called into the Rotunda every time I was in Dublin to meet up with people and catch up with what was going on in the hospital. While there was never any guarantee as to where I would end up, I would have regarded the Rotunda as home and certainly my desire was always to come back here. Then the assistant master position came up and my application was successful. Towards the end of 1996, I took up the post.

Settling back into Dublin took a bit of time. A lot of friends and family had moved to England or the United States. We had two children and one eye on the next step, but I did not know when that next step was going to happen. The social life in the hospital had changed. The tennis courts had gone and Conway's pub had closed. People were living much further out of the city, so were not staying around to socialise after work. Also, the nursing working day had changed from eight-hour to twelve-hour shifts, so they now completed their working week over three rather than five days. The midwives were not finishing work at the same time as everyone else, so going to the pub together once the work was done was not happening. There were more junior staff and they went out together, but the tight team system I had been familiar with was disappearing. Of course, I was coming back at a slightly different level and was married with children, but even with that I could sense a cultural change.

In the final year of the assistant mastership (then a senior registrar post), it was expected that the occupant would apply for a consultant position, but there were no vacancies at the Rotunda, which was where I saw myself in the long run. Peter McKenna, who was master at the time, was very good to me and allowed me to stay on. He gave me an expanded role, which was more or less a junior consultant role with my own clinical duties and more clinical autonomy, while I waited for a consultant post to come up.

***

When I returned to the Rotunda in 1996 the hospital did not have a big academic profile and the amount of research was limited but growing. Robert Harrison and the HARI unit produced clinical papers and research; Tom Clarke and Tom Matthews in neonatology also produced papers, as did pathology. Michael Darling and his successor in the mastership, Peter McKenna, brought in a research fellow to look at hypertension in pregnancy and similar projects. However, there was no expectation that everyone was going to be involved in clinical audit and research. This changed when Mike Geary was appointed master in 2002. Mike is a genuine researcher with an academic pedigree and was very supportive of research. He encouraged the junior staff and gave them the expectation that they were going to produce research.

I would not have the same academic pedigree as Mike Geary or my successor, Fergal Malone, but my strength was as a facilitator, and I could recognise the need for a solid, supportive research department. During my mastership I created a research department with a research officer and a consultant in charge of clinical audit. I was not going to lead projects, but I made sure we had people whose role was to support and promote research. It goes back to the challenge of how the Rotunda was going to be perceived as being a better hospital than others. We are not going to be better than Holles Street or the Coombe in clinical terms, because by 2009 we were all pretty much the same. However, what would differentiate us would be our ability to support staff to produce good research and write papers. That in turn would attract good candidates and good staff, and bring in research grants.

The approach worked and research in the Rotunda snowballed and is self-perpetuating. Today the Rotunda Hospital actively supports its staff in research, some of which is financed by The Rotunda Foundation. An individual's research interests are recognised as part of their contract and are honoured with allocated non-clinical time, access to a research department with a lead researcher and a statistician to help crunch the numbers, links to the RCSI for academic back-up, and, most importantly, a large source of clinical data based on the numbers of patients going through the hospital. Staff members may use their non-clinical time on a formal or informal basis, allowing them to take up a senior lectureship post. Of course, if there is a clinical crisis, they would drop everything to help as part of the supportive collegiate environment.

***

By the late 1990s the international training focus in the Rotunda began shifting towards the American model of training. The British system quietly fell out of favour following a change in the way it was structured; in Ireland there was a recognition that it was probably not quite as good or as well-run as it had been. At the same time there was a move towards more subspecialist training, the fellowship training model, which is a higher level of training and fits better with the American model. The doctors who apply for a fellowship are close to the end of their SpR training rotation and are moving towards a consultancy position. In the past fifteen years or so, several of our consultants have trained through the American system and have links to hospitals there;

in turn they have created rotations for younger doctors, thus providing greater opportunities. A doctor who has been on an obstetrics and gynaecology fellowship in the States and who wishes to continue their career in Ireland would expect to apply to one of the big four teaching and training maternity units in the country – Rotunda, Coombe, Holles Street or Cork University Hospital – where they can practise in a subspecialist service.

Fergal Malone, who succeeded me as master in 2016, has extensive connections with American university hospitals and is very much an advocate of the US fellowship training system. He completed residency training in obstetrics and gynaecology, followed by fellowship training in maternal-foetal medicine at Tufts-New England Medical Center in Boston. He worked in Columbia University in New York, where he was responsible for world-class research developments in obstetric ultrasound, prenatal diagnosis, and maternal-foetal medicine, and he directed the National Institutes of Health Maternal-Fetal Medicine Units Research Network in New York.

Fergal joined the Rotunda during Mike Geary's mastership in 2005 and was appointed Chairman of the Department of Obstetrics and Gynaecology at the RCSI based in the Rotunda. Research is one of his big strengths and, with a very strong pedigree and a great track record, he pushed the research agenda. He has been pivotal in putting together research in foetal medicine in the Rotunda – scanning, diagnostics, intervention and everything from identification of abnormalities to treating and intervening in some situations. It is a subspecialism all of its own and is very busy. The service spends a lot of time identifying and monitoring abnormalities and deciding what the best course of action is in those scenarios. For example, twin to twin transfusion would have been a cause of death for many twins in the past. Giving blood transfusions to babies in utero has saved many of those pregnancies. They are not common events, perhaps one every couple of weeks, but it is only part of what the foetal medicine service does.

Nationally, Fergal pulled together a research group, the Perinatal Ireland research consortium, that links seven maternity hospitals across the island of Ireland. Together that group of hospitals delivers at least half of the babies in Ireland. When all of their data is combined, it can match and supersede the best in the world. And when projects draw on that data, the numbers are so big that the research attracts great attention. The consortium presents regularly at the big meetings in America and elsewhere, and people really look forward to seeing what comes out of the Irish research system. It has put Ireland on the map when it comes to international research in obstetrics.

With the connections and reputation in place, most of our trainees in foetal medicine who are more than halfway through their postgraduate training have had the opportunity to undertake a rotation in the United States. There is a two-year programme with one year in the Rotunda and one in Colombia University in New York. It is extremely competitive to get on to and is very prestigious. Although now we are in a situation where we can do a lot of the training here, one should not underestimate the value of moving around from one place to another and working with different people and seeing different techniques and working within a different system.

With a few notable exceptions, most obstetricians who become consultants in Ireland will have spent time abroad, in Britain or more recently in the United States. People are returning to Ireland extraordinarily well trained and skilled in very particular areas. However, the American fellowship training system is very much designed for subspecialisation; one would do a short general training before doing an intensive fellowship or subspecialist training. This approach turns them into experts in a very narrow field quite quickly. That works easily in the United States because there might be 100 obstetrics and gynaecology consultants in a given hospital covering all areas of the specialty. In that situation you can afford to have experts working in a very narrow area and that is all that is required of them. The Irish system is designed differently and the development of subspecialisation within obstetrics and gynaecology has led to several pressing issues with regard to recruitment.

In most of our hospitals the expectation is that the work is more general; one may have a specialist interest but the general work has to be done as well. In the bigger maternity hospitals where there are more consultants it is possible to accommodate some specialist work, but everyone still needs to do the general work. Today, about a third of our consultants have done subspecialist training abroad. When they return to us, understandably they want to continue to develop their subspecialisation. The downside of this is that they are no longer being trained as generalists and, as a result, would prefer to concentrate on the higher-risk specialist clinics than do general work such as that in the low-risk antenatal clinics. This can mean that jobs at the same level are not equal. In the past we had a much smaller number of consultants; everyone was a general obstetrician and gynaecologist, perhaps with a subspecialist interest, and they took their fair share of the general workload. A balance is necessary between the two. We need to remember we have to train obstetricians and gynaecologists for all nineteen units and not just the units looking after the higher risk patients.

5

OBSTETRICS IN DUBLIN: A HISTORICAL PERSPECTIVE

● ● ● ● ● ● ● ● ●

In 2021 the three Dublin maternity hospitals, the Rotunda, the Coombe and Holles Street, are broadly similar in terms of activity levels and outcomes, and between us we deliver about 40 per cent of the mothers in Ireland. Together we provide clinical leadership in maternity and gynaecology services in the country, and act as a focus for research and audit in women's health. But this was not always the case and for many years the hospitals had different approaches, especially during the mid to late twentieth century when Catholic Church teachings had a powerful influence on obstetrical practice in Ireland. Although the Rotunda's history is rooted in the philanthropy of establishment Dublin in the eighteenth century, it is not a Protestant hospital and from the beginning the vast majority of its patients have been Roman Catholic. It is fair to say that although we were still restricted by law, we would have had the more liberal ethos that is associated with the Church of Ireland. Holles Street, on the other hand, developed very close ties with the Catholic Church when its governance was changed in 1936, and successive Holles Street masters made their allegiance to Catholic teachings very clear.[1] The Coombe was somewhere in the middle. The differences between the three maternity hospitals became evident in recent reports into some of the clinical practices of the twentieth century.

A factor that locked these different approaches into place in the twentieth century was the allegiance that consultants had to one hospital or another. Doctors tended to establish a close association with the hospital they did their early training in, so by the time they reached consultant level, they were fully imbued with the ethos of that hospital. By the late 1990s, however, a younger generation of consultants who had studied abroad was moving up through the system. In 1999 I spent the year as assistant master to Holles Street Hospital as part of the first ever rotation between the Rotunda and Holles Street. While there was still a certain amount of holding on to the old ways, change was definitely on the horizon and coming quite quickly.

***

The origins of many of the voluntary hospitals in Ireland had associations with religious organisations. They were established to help people living in the cities where poverty, crowded tenements and poor sanitation contributed to a range of diseases such as smallpox, typhoid, measles, diphtheria, whooping cough, scarlet fever, diarrhoea and tuberculosis.[2] There was no public health care or welfare system and those who could afford to be were treated in their own homes. The earlier hospitals were founded by surgeons, doctors and philanthropic individuals, who often invited influential citizens and prominent clergymen to sit on their boards in order to generate much needed support. Following Catholic Emancipation in 1829, several of our major hospitals were established by women and these included St Vincent's Hospital, founded by the Sisters of Charity in 1834, the Mercy Hospital in Cork founded by the Sisters of Mercy in 1857, and the Mater in Dublin, also a Sisters of Mercy hospital which opened in 1861. For young doctors the network of hospitals provided opportunities to develop their skills and knowledge, and they moved around, establishing professional networks that saw Irish hospitals and medical science flourish in the nineteenth century.

In the 1820s the Rotunda was the only maternity hospital in Dublin and it was turning patients away. The Coombe Hospital, a general hospital, was set up in 1823 by John Kirby, who owned a private medical school. In 1826 he opened a large ward for maternity patients. Three years later the hospital became a dedicated maternity hospital with four wards, one of which was a paying ward. Adopting the Rotunda's approach to management, a master was appointed. The Coombe Lying-In Hospital was moved to its current Cork Street location in 1967 and was renamed the Coombe Women and Children's University Hospital.[3]

Holles Street was established in 1884 by its first master, William Roe, but it ran at a loss and was closed in 1893. The following year it was reopened in new, larger premises with assistance from Dublin's lord mayor.[4] It received a Royal Charter in 1903. In 1936 the charter was amended and the governance of the hospital was altered; the new board now included the Catholic Archbishop of Dublin or his representative.

At the end of the nineteenth century and into the twentieth century, private nursing homes attached to voluntary hospitals became increasingly popular with the middle classes, who sought a higher

81

standard of treatment rather than risk a problem with a home birth. As the nursing homes were phased out, Mount Carmel Hospital, which was opened in 1950, became the main provider of private maternity care. Meanwhile the private and semi-private services in the three major maternity hospitals became more popular and provided the hospitals with an additional income stream.

The religious associations of the three hospitals were scrutinised as part of the Independent Review Group chaired by Catherine Day and the representatives of religious bodies on their boards were listed in its report in 2019.[5] In the case of the Rotunda, the ex-officio members of the Board of Governors include the Church of Ireland Archbishop of Armagh, the Church of Ireland Archbishop of Dublin, the Dean of St Patrick's and the Archdeacon of St Patrick's. In recent times, the only one of these members who took an active role in the board meetings was Gordon Linney, Archdeacon of St Patrick's from 1988 to 1994, and he remained on the board for many years after that. The controversy over the transfer of Holles Street to a site owned by St Vincent's Hospital with strong associations with the Sisters of Charity, and the potential influence of the Catholic Church on the delivery of services in the maternity hospital, is still unresolved at the time of writing.

***

I am from a mixed background; my father was Church of Ireland and my mother was from a Roman Catholic family. When I was young, religion was not an issue for me. And when do you recognise that your religion is different from other people's? In the Church of Ireland, we grew up in a community, went to a Church of Ireland national school, played football for our national school or for the parish, and generally went to a feeder secondary school which was usually a non-denominational school. We played in the same badminton club and the same tennis club, and were in cubs and scouts; that was just being part of the community we grew up in. It was only when I went to The High School, a secondary level college in Rathgar, that I became aware of other religions. There was quite a strong Jewish community in the area so there were quite a few Jewish boys and girls in the school. There were also a few Roman Catholic children. I cannot remember when my parents told me about the difficulties they had had when they were getting married. It did not really impact me in any way until Cathy and myself got married in 1988; Cathy was Roman Catholic and we were not allowed to get married in her parish as the priest refused to give us permission.

When I started working in the Rotunda as an SHO in 1989, the differences between the Rotunda and Holles Street were still pronounced, especially with regard to fertility, sterilisation and the use of caesarean section; the Rotunda took a more liberal approach than Holles Street on each of these matters. These differences were entrenched by medical staff remaining associated with one or other hospital for their entire professional careers. Each of the three Dublin maternity hospitals would take someone in at SHO level and train them in their way of doing things. The person may have gone away and come back at a more senior level, but they would still have been very much the hospital's own person. So, when I moved to Holles Street as assistant master for one year on the rotation between the two hospitals, I was the first non-Holles-Street-trained obstetrician to be appointed to a relatively senior position in that hospital.

The rotation between the Rotunda and Holles Street was the first formal rotation between any two hospitals at a senior registrar level in the country. It came about because of a recognition that we needed more structure in the training of obstetricians and that training rotations were a way to do it. It was also recognised that it was no longer practical to take someone into a hospital as a junior doctor, train them from start to finish, and mould them in an individual hospital's particular way. Peter McKenna and Declan Keane, masters of the Rotunda and Holles Street respectively, arranged the rotation. Two people, one from each hospital, were appointed to the three-year assistant master post. The idea was that each started in their own hospital, moved for the second year to the other hospital, and returned to their own hospital for the third year. I was to swap with Laurence Impey. However, at the end of the first year, Laurence got a consultant post in Oxford. His rotation was taken up by Mike Geary, who wanted to do his first year in Holles Street so I did my second year in the Rotunda, then we swapped for my third year.

In 1999 the assistant master post was still close to the traditional model, where the incumbent was a senior non-consultant hospital doctor who played quite an important role within the hospital. As assistant master I was responsible for running the rota for the non-consultant hospital doctors, and for much of the day-to-day oversight of obstetrics for public patients in the hospital, which was a fairly substantial clinical role. I worked closely with the consultants and especially with the master, who oversaw everything that I did. Holles Street was still quite regimented and they had their way of doing things based on Kieran O'Driscoll's active management of labour.

The master, Declan Keane, was very much in the tradition of Holles Street. A UCD graduate, he was only a year older than myself (I played rugby against him at school). When he attended the hospital's monthly meetings to talk about the figures and the statistics, all of the Holles

Street ex-masters would have been in attendance; if he was doing anything of which they disapproved, such as indicating a rise in the caesarean section rate, he would have had some explaining to do. The ex-masters were formidable characters and were absolutely convinced that their way was the right way. Yet while there was still a certain amount of holding on to the old ways, a younger generation of consultants was working with new ideas and new ways of doing things. Even during my one year there, I could see changes happening quite quickly.

I was welcomed by the hospital staff. There was an institutional, convent-like sense to the hospital, but also a warm, family atmosphere, not unlike the Rotunda. Fairly early on I picked up on an initial distrust of my training. I also encountered the rigidity of the thinking that was prevalent in the hospital at that time. The main difference that I came across was in relation to how far we would let a pregnancy continue. For quite some time in the Rotunda we had a system in place where women were not allowed to go too far over their due date and therefore we would have had a higher induction rate for post-date pregnancies. If you induce someone there is a much higher chance that they will need a caesarean section. My own policy at that stage would have been ten days maximum.

In Holles Street their policy was to allow women to go overdue for much longer and we were not allowed to induce people with post-dates earlier than about fourteen days. I found that difficult, because there is plenty of evidence to support the fact that the longer the pregnancy goes on the more likely there are going to be problems either with foetal distress or stillbirth. Based on my years of experience, I had developed parameters that I was happy to work within, but I was suddenly plunged into a situation where I was being asked to work outside those parameters. I found myself a bit lost as to what happened next. Where did one go? Should I create another set of parameters that I would be happy to work within? I found it quite stressful and it took me a while to find a way around the system.

The first major issue I came up against was on one of my first nights on call. I was asked by a midwife to do a scalp pH on a patient who was fully dilated; a scalp pH is to take a small blood sample from the baby's scalp and run it through a machine to check the baby's oxygen levels. I thought that this was unusual: normally that is an obstetric decision rather than a midwifery decision. The trace was not particularly good, nor was the foetal monitoring particularly good or reassuring. So I told the sister that the patient needed to be delivered. The sister insisted that in this situation the hospital normally did a scalp pH. I, in turn, insisted that the patient needed to be delivered. The patient was a private patient of one of the consultants. I went to do something else while the sister phoned the consultant and, as I came back into the office, I heard her saying to the consultant that Dr Coulter Smith was refusing to do a pH on this lady and asking what to do. I asked to speak to the consultant and I explained to him the situation, saying that the patient needed to be delivered and if he didn't want to come in and do it, then I was happy to do it. The consultant asked me to do a scalp pH just to keep the peace. I refused, reiterating that the patient needed to be delivered now. He came in and delivered her. The baby had meconium aspiration and had to go straight to the neonatal unit. After a rocky few days in neonatal intensive care, the baby went back to the mother and was fine in the long run.

My decision that the patient needed to be delivered was the right one. It was also a game changer in terms of my relationship with the labour ward midwives. I was proven right in the choice I had made. Until then, because I had come from the Rotunda, there would not have been the same degree of trust in my decisions. But after that incident they realised that maybe I did have some idea of what I was talking about and that perhaps they should listen to me the next time. At the same time, I respected the fact that they did things differently and were very committed to their way. What it taught me is that you cannot pigeonhole anyone; obstetrics is a very individual thing and you cannot make a definite plan for everybody. You have to roll with situations and adapt to the individual patient's circumstances.

I did not run into any more problems after that. I settled in and was fully accepted. I loved my time there. There was a real sense of everyone pulling in the same direction, and a very strong sense of loyalty to the hospital similar to that in the Rotunda. I enjoyed being part of this very committed group of professionals who had a great desire to achieve.

The senior registrar rotation between the Rotunda and Holles Street only ran for a few years. What came fairly quickly after that was the structured SpR training system and for five years the young doctors would go from hospital to hospital. Then the Institution of Obstetrics and Gynaecologists took on the role of appointing trainees within hospitals and with that came the centralised process of appointing registrars. The assistant mastership position still exists, but it has changed over the course of the last twenty or so years. In the past the position would have been filled by someone who specifically applied for the job as in my case; the person would have pretty much completed their training and was waiting in the wings for a consultant post. Now the assistant master is the most senior SpR on a particular six month or year-long rotation and they do not apply specifically for the role, nor are they interviewed for it. While it is still a senior registrar position, it is not as high-ranking a post as it was. The assistant masters run the rota for the junior doctors, have a greater input in terms of management and administration, and get involved in hospital committees and clinical risk, and feedback on clinical risk to the juniors.

***

The historical difference in the ethos of the Rotunda and Holles Street was evident in their approach to caesarean sections. In the twentieth century Irish obstetrical practice was heavily influenced by certain religious principles and constrained within a legislative framework that ensured conformity to those principles. Artificial contraception had been banned by the Criminal Law Amendment Act of 1935 and it was illegal for doctors to provide information about it.[6] This led to Ireland's birth rate being one of the highest in Europe, with many women delivering eight or more babies.[7] Sterilisation to prevent conception was not permitted except where there was a serious danger to the woman.

Throughout history caesarean sections were used in cases of pelvic disproportion or obstructed birth, but most of the women and babies died. With the development of anaesthesia in the mid-nineteenth century, survival became possible. The first successful caesarean section in Ireland was reported by the master of the Rotunda, Arthur Macan, in 1889.[8] With safe anaesthesia and good success with the procedure, caesarean sections soon became a viable option for an obstructed delivery.

In the early twentieth century, the Rotunda had a 0.09 incident rate of caesarean sections, or 13 out of 13,924 deliveries from 1903 to 1910.[9] By 1944 that rate had risen to 2.28 per cent. Over in Holles Street, Dr Horne in 1902 recommended that caesarean sections should be performed early in labour, pointing out that delay before doing a caesarean section was a grave error.[10] However, the attitude then shifted and for much of the twentieth century every effort was made to avoid performing caesarean sections in Holles Street.

When I started in the Rotunda in 1989, we were well out of the era when women died as a result of complications from caesarean sections. Anaesthesia associated with operative obstetrics had improved dramatically and was a whole lot safer. In the Rotunda this was down to anaesthetic consultants Bill Blunnie and Jim Gardner, both of whom were jointly appointed with the Mater Hospital. There were still consultants in the Rotunda – like Mike Darling and George Henry – who had trained and worked at a time when caesarean sections rates were in single figures and there would have been a significant risk to the mother. By the time I came along, the surgical procedure was well established and improving all of the time, but we still had to justify why we had done that intervention at a weekly caesarean section meetings. Every caesarean section that had been done during the previous week was reviewed at those meetings and the obstetrician responsible had to justify and explain it; if I had done one when on call, the spotlight was on me and I had to defend it.

In 1989, at the first meeting of RAMI that I attended, there was plenty of discussion about caesarean section rates. The emphasis in Holles Street was still on achieving vaginal deliveries and it was clearly a badge of honour on their part that they had the lowest caesarean rate in the country. In the Rotunda we were willing to have a higher intervention rate for better outcomes. The Coombe traditionally had a caesarean rate that was behind ours but always higher than Holles Street.

The determination on the part of Holles Street to have a low caesarean section rate seemed to have peaked in the mid-twentieth century under Masters Alex Spain (1942–48) and Arthur Barry (1949–55). Both held strong Catholic beliefs and were concerned that an obstetrician might perform a sterilisation or hysterectomy during a caesarean section to help the patient avoid further pregnancies. Spain described sterilisation for contraceptive purposes as mutilation.[11] But many obstetricians at this time were conflicted. Women, often in poor health, were turning up for their tenth or fifteenth or even twentieth delivery. Repeated obstetric anaesthesia and caesarean sections were risky for women where a vaginal delivery was not possible; there was a fair chance they were going to die either from complications of the anaesthetic, from complications of infection or from bleeding. Restrained by legislation, there was little the obstetricians could legally do to help them control their fertility, so achieving a vaginal delivery on the first birth was preferred, even if it was carried through at some cost to the woman.

Rotunda obstetrician Michael Solomons described the situations facing the medical teams on a regular basis in the 1940s. Michael, the son of Rotunda master Bethel Solomons, began his career with the Rotunda as a student in 1939. He worked on the District service for a while and was clinical clerk for six months in 1943. He described the homes in which his patients lived in and around the Rotunda as being in dilapidated Georgian buildings with no electricity or running water, primitive toilet facilities, a communal tap on the ground floor, peeling paint, leaking ceilings and poor waste facilities. Tuberculosis and gastroenteritis were common, as were malnutrition and anaemia. During this time as clinical clerk, the students under his management attended 785 home deliveries of which ninety-three were to women pregnant for at least the tenth time. Fourteen of these women were giving birth for the fourteenth time and one woman was admitted to hospital miscarrying on her twenty-first pregnancy.[12] He described how a twenty-six-year-old woman with high blood pressure on her sixth pregnancy went blind, only to return pregnant again the following year.[13] He also cited a colleague who delivered a baby with a Guinness bottle cap stuck on its head; the mother had used it in a failed attempt to avoid conception.[14] Years later Solomons was instrumental in introducing family planning to Ireland.

Symphysiotomy is an age-old surgical procedure, which enlarges the mother's pelvis during labour to facilitate the delivery of the baby more easily. The first successful symphysiotomy was described in France in 1777, and although it was undertaken without anaesthetic or knowledge of infection, it was a major advance in managing breech and otherwise obstructed deliveries.[15] Symphysiotomy first made its appearance in Irish medical literature in 1897, by which time anaesthetic and antiseptic procedures were in place. Pubiotomy, which involved the division of the pubic bone for severe cases of obstructed delivery, was possible from 1902 when the right equipment became available. However, it was seldom used in the Rotunda.[16]

As caesarean sections became more feasible in the early twentieth century, the need for symphysiotomy dropped off and by the 1940s it was rarely used in Britain or Europe. The Rotunda preferred the caesarean section as a solution to obstructed labour. The masters, especially Eric W.L. Thompson (known as Bill), master from 1952 to 1959, disliked symphysiotomy as it could cause lifelong pelvic instability. However, symphysiotomy was going through a revival in other Irish hospitals, notably Holles Street under the masterships of Spain and Barry.[17]

Looking at the annual reports of the three Dublin maternity hospitals, evidence suggests that the Holles Street and the Coombe were pro-symphysiotomy and anti-caesarean section. At the height of its use in Dublin, from the mid-1940s to the mid-1950s, symphysiotomy accounted for 0.4 per cent of total deliveries at the Coombe and 0.34

per cent at Holles Street.[18] During the same period the Rotunda did none most years and very few in the other years, but its caesarean rate increased from 1.1 to 4.6 per cent and remained on a steady upward trajectory. At the time symphysiotomy was statistically a safer procedure than caesarean section, with no maternal deaths recorded as opposed to two annually with caesareans. Symphysiotomy was used in other maternity units, most notably in Our Lady of Lourdes in Drogheda, where they continued to use the procedure until 1984.[19]

Although symphysiotomy was statistically an exceptional procedure, the Irish approach came under fire from invited British obstetricians in the mid-twentieth century. At the 1951 RAMI meeting to discuss the annual reports, the discussion revolved around the conservative obstetrical environment in Dublin and explicit links were made to religious beliefs; obstetricians even quoted the Bible at each other. It was recognised that the drive to get the baby out vaginally was partly coming from a religious ethos; they would use symphysiotomy to ensure that the woman's next delivery would be a vaginal birth. The visiting obstetrician, Professor Chassar Moir, spoke, stating that he viewed the Irish obstetricians' determination to push for vaginal deliveries in Dublin with some anxiety. He had no objection to symphysiotomy in cases of disproportion where absolutely necessary, but asked, 'Is it then your policy to sacrifice the firstborn baby and to use its dead or dying body as nothing more than a battering ram to stretch its mother's pelvis in the hope that subsequent brothers and sisters may thereby have (possibly) an easier entrance into this world?'[20]

In 2014, during my mastership, an investigation into twentieth-century use of symphysiotomy in Irish maternity hospitals was published. The subject had been raised in the early twenty-first century when the long-term effects of the procedure on some women were brought to public attention. It was only then that people realised how common it had been and there were calls upon successive ministers for health to hold an inquiry. At the Rotunda a number of women had come forward who had had a symphysiotomy. Peter McKenna, the master, arranged for the women to be examined by people from obstetrics, orthopaedics and urology. There were few issues identified in that group.

Professor Oonagh Walsh of Glasgow Caledonian University produced the *Report on Symphysiotomy in Ireland, 1944–1984* for Minister for Health James Reilly. During the course of her investigations, she examined the complex interaction of medical, socio-religious and cultural factors around the procedure. It was not a huge issue for the Rotunda because we had had so few cases. It was, however, a big issue for Holles Street and for Our Lady of Lourdes Hospital in Drogheda. It is evident from Professor Walsh's report that there are some women with long-term problems associated with symphysiotomy. But for me working in a busy gynaecology clinic for twenty-five years, I have never come across someone who had pelvic floor concerns or issues related to a symphysiotomy.

***

By the 1960s caesarean sections were on the rise in Irish maternity hospitals and units, but Holles Street, true to its ethos and its determination to avoid the procedure, sought a new way of dealing with obstructed births. Kieran O'Driscoll, master from 1963 to 1969, developed the active management of labour (AML), a group of interventions initially devised to shorten labour in first-time mothers and in this way avoid the use of symphysiotomy in an obstructed birth as well as keep caesarean section rates low.[21] AML is about accurate diagnosis of labour with one midwife supporting the patient during labour. In many ways it is a good, sensible approach on when and how to intervene in order to keep labour moving in the right direction. If a patient's labour is shortened appropriately, less intervention may be required because the mother won't develop a temperature, and the baby won't become distressed and end up having to be delivered in an emergency situation by caesarean section. Holles Street was very good at this. The midwives were invested in it; having a good midwife to look after the mother might mean that medics would not have to intervene. AML helped to reduce the incidence of abnormal labour and helped to make symphysiotomy obsolete except in rare emergencies.[22]

Kieran O'Driscoll wrote a manual on AML that became a standard textbook in the management of labour internationally. The fourth edition was published in 2003. Many people would regard AML as medicalisation of a normal process, but Kieran O'Driscoll would have referred to this as keeping things normal. I think there is still some good stuff in there; one-on-one support for a woman in labour and making sure she is relaxed and well looked after is all very positive. But some of it is now outdated and where it probably fell down was in striving at all costs for a vaginal delivery in the first pregnancy; one size was expected to fit all and if you were a first-time mother, this was the way the hospital did things and it was not going to change for anyone. There is a cost in relation to reluctance to intervene and a reluctance to do a caesarean section. As a result, there will be damaged babies and higher numbers of HIE cases, and I think the zealots of AML maybe gave the approach a slightly bad name because of that. In the Rotunda we followed some of those principles, but we were a bit more liberal with others and we did not call it active management of labour.

Even as late as 1999, when I arrived on my rotation, keeping the caesarean section low was still the Holles Street way, and many of their staff were very proud of their very low section rates. They would also have been very aware that the Rotunda had a more liberal approach and they may have been nervous that I was going to bring that influence with me. Initially, I found their rigid thinking difficult, but there were lots of good things associated with it and I learned how to manage.

In recent times training rotations for young trainee doctors move them from unit to unit each year and consequently they do not become moulded in the customs of one institution. They learn different ways of doing things, which they bring to wherever they are appointed. It is no longer possible to have a regimented style of training any more. Plus we are now living in an age where there are national and international guidelines for just about everything, so it is almost impossible to be too different. But the fact that the book on AML was written in and came from Dublin, where we have a very strong history and culture of reporting our data annually, enabled the active management story to be spread worldwide. Obstetricians who wanted to keep their caesarean sections rates low looked to Dublin, studied the evidence for AML in the annual reports on a rolling basis, and adopted AML in part or in whole. As a result Dublin developed a very strong reputation for obstetric management.

Today the rates of caesarean sections in Irish maternity hospitals are higher and are mostly on a par with each other, but with a few exceptions. The change in thinking towards caesarean sections probably started in the 1990s, when it was clear that the procedure was much safer than it used to be thanks to antibiotics and regional anaesthesia. Now, in the Rotunda, the question is more likely to be why we did not do a caesarean section in particular circumstances rather than why we did do one. The caesarean section weekly meetings have been replaced with the cardiotocography (CTG) meeting, which is a teaching meeting around interpreting the results of the baby's heartbeat in labour and when to intervene.

We monitor our caesarean section rates closely and audit the rate weekly using the Robson criteria. One of the categories that will influence future caesarean section rates concerns the management of women who had a previous section. It has always been known that you could go back to a vaginal birth after a caesarean (VBAC), but the pendulum has been swinging too far in the opposite direction. In the Rotunda we are working to balance this by being proactive and encouraging VBAC in appropriate cases. For some women it is not appropriate to have a vaginal birth because of the situation of their first birth, but the team has the responsibility to identify women who have had caesarean sections in the past and who may be suitable for a vaginal birth for a subsequent labour. Obstetricians, midwives, physiotherapists and others are involved in the assessment about whether a patient might be supported to have a vaginal birth. Midwives and obstetricians talk to the women and find out if they are amenable to trying a vaginal birth. Many women are keen to try and there is no need to talk them around, but others will have made up their minds and want a caesarean section. If potential VBAC cases are selected and managed well, it is possible to achieve vaginal delivery in 60 to 70 per cent of patients if they go into labour spontaneously. It is one group of patients where we can make a difference; it takes time and effort to try for the less complicated outcome, so the hospital has to be motivated to support the pregnant woman in her choice for a VBAC.

During my time as master, we did try to control the caesarean section rate as much as we could. I also believed that VBAC was an important issue and I encouraged it. The caesarean section rate stayed fairly constant during my mastership, rising only two or three per cent, and the section rate for women who had had previous sections was lower. But given the commitment and time involved in encouraging a vaginal birth where a potential complication has been identified, it is not surprising that some maternity units decide to go straight for the caesarean section. Nationally this is pushing up caesarean rates, especially in HSE hospitals. Cavan Hospital, which is in our RCSI Hospital Group, is a good example where the caesarean section rate is now nearly fifty per cent because they will not take any risks. And if a patient has already had a caesarean birth, she will be counselled to have another on subsequent births. Some will argue that there is nothing wrong with that, but it means that there is an extraordinarily high section rate with associated complications and issues for subsequent pregnancies.

***

Today the three Dublin maternity hospitals, the Rotunda, the Coombe and Holles Street, have formed their own joint maternities committee with an independent chairperson. Generally voluntary hospitals are happy to work together on clinical matters but tend to keep their management to themselves, so this was an unusual move. The fact that the three hospitals are broadly similar in terms of their activities and their level of activity is hugely helpful and supportive. They act as a powerful lobby and can deal with the very real issues that relate exclusively to the Dublin maternity hospitals. Each month four people from each hospital, the master, the chair of the board, the secretary manager and the director of midwifery, meet. There is a rolling agenda addressing issues that we are all facing. This has been going on for some time, certainly since the 1990s, and it is a useful forum. Services and other detailed matters might be discussed over lunch, but this forum is for discussion on how we might handle common issues of significance. We have all been put under pressure by the state health authorities at various times to do something or to adopt something or react to something and this joint meeting is a very good way of ensuring that each hospital knows that it is not on its own and that we can all approach concerns in the same way, providing support and giving some strength in numbers.

6

PROMOTING INNOVATION

● ● ● ● ● ● ● ● ●

The Rotunda Hospital's governance structure is designed to facilitate innovation, change, learning and research, and ever since our foundation we have developed new services as the need arises. The Board of Governors together with the master and the executive management team plan strategically. They oversee activity, examine outcomes, put key performance indicators (KPIs) in place and identify the need for new service developments that may be required. Our regular reporting, auditing and analysis, together with our KPIs, help us identify what we need to do to make improvements or to address issues. Our independence then gives us flexibility, freedom to do things that are outside the box and to respond rapidly to evolving situations. We have small but significant amounts of money that come from our own funding sources and are under our control. Mostly, establishing a new service requires a reallocation of existing resources, but sometimes a new post is created or new equipment acquired for a service to be set up.

In 2000, at the end of my rotation, I returned to the Rotunda from Holles Street and participated in the continued development of a service that had been created due to demand. At the time I was more than ready for a consultant post, but there were no vacancies so I continued in a senior registrar position. Peter McKenna, now in the sixth year of his mastership, gave me the made-up title of 'first assistant to the master' and additional responsibilities that allowed me to act as a junior consultant but under the master's wing. I was given a gynaecology clinic, an operating list and a lot of clinical autonomy. At the same time I was appointed the clinical lead in the fairly new clinic that had been set up to care for patients with infectious diseases. Just as I took over, the scope of this clinic had to be expanded to look after an influx of women from sub-Saharan Africa who were arriving on a weekly basis at Dublin airport heavily pregnant and with unknown previous histories. This was a classic instance of how a voluntary hospital can respond swiftly to an unanticipated situation in a way that the HSE hospitals would find much more difficult.

***

The evolution of the Rotunda is a history of continuous development, from the establishment of significant new services such as gynaecology, neonatology and the medical social services, to the creation of specialist clinics for patients with anaemia, diabetes, infectious disease, haematology and many other issues, as well as additional services such as family planning, infertility and sterilisation. The master has always been responsible for ensuring that patient needs are identified and new services introduced. In the early days when the hospital was not so complex, the need for a new service could be obvious, although the resources may have been difficult to come by. Our first pathology department, for example, was opened by Richard Dancer Purefoy in

1902 at his own expense. It flourished until lack of funds closed it down at the end of the First World War. For a number of years, the testing of specimens was outsourced to the RCSI. In 1926 Bethel Solomons reopened the laboratory.

The hospital attracted exceptional pathologists including the serologist Professor Hans Sachs in 1941. Professor Sachs (1877–1945) was a distinguished German Jewish refugee who had been the Director of the Institute of Cancer Research at Heidelberg and was associated with developments in immunology. While in the Rotunda, he investigated the distribution of blood groups in Ireland and became the first person to perform Rhesus blood group typing in the country. Arising from his work, determining the Rhesus group was introduced into the antenatal routine of the Rotunda.[1] He was also known for his work on the diagnosis of syphilis;[2] in 1943–44, 1,265 women had their blood tested and ninety-two received anti-syphilitic treatment.[3] The pathology department continues to attract exceptional people right up to today, such as consultant microbiologist Richard Drew, who was appointed in 2014 during my time as master. Richard is very forward-thinking and very keen on early pick-up and diagnosis of infection in general. When Covid-19 became an issue in 2020, he already had in place the equipment and a system to allow us to develop a test so we could get answers quickly. Within four weeks of the outbreak, we were testing patients for the virus inhouse.

Another historical development in the Rotunda worth noting at this point was the establishment of the medical social work department. Although it is not clinical and is now a department within a department, it supports our specialist clinics, including, for example, the infectious diseases clinic. The social work department was set up in 1934 when a trained almoner was appointed.[4] Originally this position was to ascertain whether a patient was capable of paying a portion of the fees for treatment. However, most of our patients at that time were local women, many living in terrible conditions, and the almoner's work became more about helping them with social issues. The Rotunda almoners often negotiated with the housing section of Dublin Corporation and with other agencies to help with shelter and basic nourishment; they also had access to their own Samaritan Fund. Eleanor Holmes, who was head medical social worker from 1954 to 1987, wrote of a mother in 1942 who became pregnant for the twenty-first time. Fifteen of her children were alive, three had died and she had had two miscarriages; one of her children had rickets. She had fainted in the streets and was said to be starving, which is why she was referred to the almoner. Her husband was unemployed, depressed and demoralised; the children had no shoes, minimal clothing and were living in one room; and the patient had severe anaemia and was in despair. The almoner coordinated a number of agencies including St John Ambulance, which helped with dinners, the Infant Aid Society, which supplied milk for the children, and the Rotunda Samaritan, which provided further assistance. Dublin Corporation rehoused the family in Cabra.[5] Arising from an endless series of cases like this, the hospital established an Anaemia Clinic in 1953 under consultant general physician Dr Peter Gatenby. He provided medical recommendations for rehousing patients with poor nutrition and poor home conditions. His recommendations supplemented the almoner's letters to the housing authorities.

Up to 1954 the social workers in the Rotunda asked to see marriage certificates of all public patients before they were booked in. This was prompted by concern about any irregular circumstances that might compromise the safety of the infant, moral or otherwise. Nevertheless, single women were admitted and shared the wards with the married women. This caused some difficulties for the unmarried women, and from 1954 the almoners kept a supply of cheap wedding rings from Woolworths for their use. Every woman was given the prefix Mrs and everyone was addressed by that title rather than by first name. Although the almoners were criticised for encouraging subterfuge and dishonesty, they carried on, even arranging for male relatives to visit unmarried patients in the early evening when husbands usually visited.

In 1964 almoners became known as medical social workers. From that time onwards, they have found themselves helping with a range of social issues including marriage counselling, child protection, family planning, extra marital pregnancy, bereavement, addiction issues and, in the 1980s, HIV/AIDs. Child abuse and neglect, and non-accidental injuries to children were mentioned in the social work section of the clinical report for first time in 1975. Social workers set themselves the task of early identification of at-risk mothers. The social workers linked in with external organisations such as the churches for marriage guidance, the Women's Aid Society for women in domestic violent situations and so on.

Today the medical social workers are part of a multidisciplinary team. For the medical staff, the main interaction is recognising when a patient needs support and then linking them in with the social workers. In the past, for example, I would have referred young girls who had become pregnant to get on the social housing list in order to escape their circumstances; this tends not to happen now. Although the medical workers are part of the hospital, the master would not have as much oversight of their service as they would of pathology, radiology or paediatrics, for example. As master I would have known the number of patients seen and whether the staff were coping with their workload, but otherwise it ran alongside other services.

***

The social workers were involved in the multidisciplinary team that cared for our patients in the infectious diseases clinic. When this clinic was set up, the hospital already had several specialist clinics, including one for patients with diabetes and another for those who were obese. The purpose of creating these clinics was to ensure that the women attending with specific conditions met the same medical team each time. The infectious diseases clinic came about in the late 1990s, when we had a sudden increase in the number of patients with this particular issue. Women presenting with infectious diseases had always been around, whether it was tuberculosis or syphilis. In 1985 the Rotunda commenced HIV clinical testing, but the medical social work department successfully lobbied against segregating these patients. At the same time the hospital policy concerning infectious diseases was upgraded and all medical staff were to assume that patients were carrying something. If they knew someone was positive for a highly infectious disease, they would take extra precautions, such as double gloving and wearing masks and goggles.

By the late 1990s, the situation shifted. In a short space of time we had an increased number of patients with HIV, and the master, Peter McKenna, decided that they would be cared for better if there was a dedicated group of professionals looking after their particular needs. They had risks and issues that were unique to them in their pregnancy, so it made sense to have a clinic that they could come to on a regular basis and be seen by the same group of professionals. Former master George Henry was clinical lead of the new clinic and the team included a registrar and some midwives who had a special interest in the area. Many of the women guided to the clinic had difficult lives with multiple issues, such as poor diets, poor social circumstances and maybe drug abuse. This made them prone to infectious diseases. The team got to know the patients and their problems, so every time the women came in they were provided with continuity of care and did not have to repeat themselves. The midwives devoted a lot of time to sorting out the clinical issues and being the point of contact for these women.

Of all the infectious diseases we see, HIV is the one that requires rapid testing. If a patient is HIV positive and has a high viral load but is unaware of it, there is a high risk that she will transfer the virus to the baby in utero during labour with a vaginal birth. For some of the women who are HIV positive, it is important that they have a caesarean section. The caesarean section itself is straightforward, but the baby needs to be washed down quickly afterwards. Getting to these patients early and starting them on antiviral treatment as soon as possible to get their viral loads down is a very important part of the care they get. That is why early identification and early intervention is so important in those cases. Hepatitis, syphilis and other infectious diseases are not as important in this regard.

As time went by we were able to manage those patients better. The Rotunda had been doing routine antenatal HIV testing for some years and was the first hospital to identify a need for this. When Mike Darling was master, an anonymous prevalence study was arranged. For a certain amount of time, everyone had an anonymised HIV test as part of their regular blood tests to see what the prevalence of HIV was in the population. Based on the results, HIV testing was brought in and everyone had to consent to HIV testing as part of their booking process. Introducing it was something that we thought would be more difficult than it actually was; while there was a little pushback at first, there was not as much as we anticipated. As the midwives who met the patients became more comfortable talking about the HIV test, the patients accepted it as simply one of the routine blood tests. For many years we had had to courier tests out to St James's Hospital and wait several days for the results. Now the Rotunda pathology department could do all of the HIV, hepatitis and other infectious disease testing. The in-house turnaround time was quick, probably within a day, so we could get all of the information we needed rapidly. We were the first to do this and antenatal testing for HIV was to become a national standard.

The challenge with this group of women was – and still is – to keep the HIV vertical transmission (VT) rate right down (the VT rate relates to the number of babies born who test positive for the disease). In the 1990s managing and treating women with HIV in pregnancy was relatively new and we were the first hospital in Ireland to set up this type of clinic. Auditing the outcomes, including the VT rate, was important. We would always try to get the VT rate as low as possible and we would measure ourselves against other hospitals and units, although our numbers were always greater because of where we are situated. If results from elsewhere were better, we would try to find out what they were doing that we were not. As in many areas, the Rotunda is a leader in this field, and our policies and processes in this regard were taken up by other hospitals. As new anti-viral drugs came on the market, many of our patients were involved in trials for different antiretroviral treatments. We worked closely with Jack Lambert and the infectious diseases team in the Mater Hospital to co-manage these patients. This was an important collaboration and the studies that were carried out, together with results, were presented at meetings and published in research papers. I also wrote the first guidelines in Ireland for HIV in pregnancy.

**

In the early 2000s, shortly after I took over the obstetric clinical lead of the infectious diseases clinic, there was an unforeseen influx of women from sub-Saharan Africa who were in an advanced stage of pregnancy. At the time the law was such that children born in Ireland would automatically receive Irish citizenship, and their parents were generally granted residency; this had arisen from the Good Friday Agreement in 1998. Some of the women came with HIV, hepatitis and syphilis as well as other conditions. They were arriving at Dublin Airport on flights from London and often on a Friday afternoon. The demands on our clinic suddenly grew in size and complexity. With some of them actually in labour, they were brought in a minibus to the Rotunda because we were the nearest maternity hospital to the airport. The emergency room and the labour ward became overwhelmed with all of this unplanned level of activity. We set up a triaging system to do an accurate diagnosis and to gather information as to what was going on with their pregnancy in order to provide them with the best possible care. The women who were in labour were checked in and delivered. We had no idea what had happened to them in the past; we had no idea whether they were HIV positive and no idea of what other issues they may have had. Some of them had already had a caesarean section and some had had female genital mutilation performed, so they came with social and clinical issues that mostly we did not know about or fully understand.

It became a very difficult situation and we felt we had to do something about it. So Mike Geary, who was appointed master in 2002, George Henry and myself set up a clinic in Balseskin Reception Centre near the airport. The African women were taken to Balseskin by Department of Justice staff and they met our midwives and social workers there. We triaged the women, assessed them from an obstetric point of view, ascertained whether they were HIV positive or had other infectious diseases, and assessed their risk issues. From there we organised for them to stay in Dublin if that was appropriate for their obstetric needs, or arranged for them to be sent to other hospitals around the country or on to other services. It became so busy that we made an agreement with the Coombe and Holles Street that they would take some patients after we had triaged them.

The Rotunda infectious diseases clinic coordinated the whole service for these women. We did not get paid for the service by the Department of Justice, but the Department of Health approved new jobs, including my own position, as a result of it. Obstetricians, midwives and social workers were involved in this service and we met the women for only a brief time during antenatal consultations. We were perceived as being people in authority and the women were quite often suspicious of us. With no homes to go to and no family support, the women had massive social issues. Some of them were genuine asylum seekers and coming from very difficult backgrounds and very difficult situations. Some were well educated and affluent. Many were reluctant to tell their story for fear that they might be sent back; others would tell you everything, where they were from and how they got here. Often, they had paid money to be transported to Ireland. But it was none of our business how they got here; our focus was medical and we were only dealing with them for a relatively short period of time. However, it put them on guard about how much information they were going to provide and how accurate it was. This was a challenge. In order to provide appropriate care, we needed as much accurate information as possible. We needed to know what might have happened in previous pregnancies but the more we quizzed them, the more we questioned, the more defensive they became and would not necessarily give us accurate information.

There were other issues for the women. African women are great at breastfeeding and one of the difficult things for an HIV positive woman is that she cannot do that. This was very tough on them because bottle feeding her baby suggested to her community that she was HIV positive. The midwives helped them to manage this.

In 2004 the law changed and it was no longer possible for a mother and child to get an Irish passport if the child was born in Ireland. Soon we started to see the numbers of sub-Saharan African women fall away, but they were replaced by an influx of women from eastern Europe, especially Latvia, Lithuania and Romania, as a result of the expansion of the European Union.

For a little while patients attending the infectious disease clinic would have DOI, Danger of Infection, on a large label stuck on the outside of their chart. Often patients carried their own chart around the hospital with them. It was a bit like putting a sticker on someone saying, 'I have an infection'! A group of us discussed it over lunch and the name was changed to DOVE, Danger of Viral Exposure, because it sounded nicer. The DOVE clinic continues to this day.

***

George Henry retired in 2002 and a consultancy position came up. I was the successful candidate. Becoming a consultant is a pretty enormous step. When a doctor has reached the point of being a senior registrar of good standing, the likelihood is that an appointment to a consultancy is going to happen, but where and when are the unknowns. As a consultant you are accountable, you are the boss, you practise solo and you make independent decisions that are final clinical decisions; the autonomy of a consultant is ultimate but this can be daunting. At that point I had done over ten years in training and had been a senior registrar for five years and I was quite at home in my own ability, so becoming a consultant came at the right time for me. I was delighted and relieved at the same time.

I had waited for this position. I could have applied for a job in a regional hospital maternity unit, such as Cavan, Drogheda or Wexford, but our parents and families were in Dublin and we had returned from London to work in the city. Also, I was striving to be in division one, so I was looking for a job in the Rotunda, Holles Street or the Coombe. But the Rotunda was where I wanted to be and where I saw myself. The advantage of a bigger hospital like the Rotunda is that there are more consultants around us and more people on site and available, willing and able to give advice and to help out when it is required. In a smaller unit, there may be only two or three consultants on the staff and any number of reasons why there might be no help available – someone might be on holidays, or one may not get on with another – so that culture of providing assistance and helping out may not necessarily be there. The problems associated with this are clearly highlighted in Judge Clark's 2006 report into peripartum hysterectomy in Our Lady of Lourdes Hospital in Drogheda, where Dr Michael Neary was working without support.[6] In the Rotunda, a consultant still has clinical autonomy, but if someone's outcomes are in any way unusual or if there are complications, these will be highlighted fairly quickly through regular audit meetings. We have a fairly strict way of overseeing clinical practice to the extent that any chance that someone may become an outlier is picked up before that happens. The collegiate type of atmosphere we have always had in the Rotunda is a huge advantage. Here it is not considered to be a sign of weakness for a consultant to say that they have a difficult situation and to ask others for ideas on what they might do.

***

Today the need for new services or investment in new equipment or some other innovation continues to arise. A need may be raised at one of our regular meetings, someone may come back from abroad with new information, or someone who has worked elsewhere realises that we could manage a little bit better in the Rotunda if we had a special clinic looking after particular patients. The ability to examine these ideas and address these needs is still integral to the management and governance structure of voluntary hospitals like the Rotunda.

It was gratifying to see that this flexibility was specifically recognised in the 2019 report by Catherine Day and the IRG on voluntary hospitals. The IRG report identifies as one of the added values of the voluntary hospitals their 'capacity to innovate, testing new ideas and constantly updating to improve patient/service user care'.[7] The report also noted, 'There was widespread agreement that the voluntary sector brings innovation, flexibility, independence and strong commitment to delivery of health and social care. This is consistent with findings [with voluntary hospitals] in other countries.'[8]

However, Day also points out that state funding to the voluntary hospitals 'does not allow for any innovation or reform or piloting of new ideas and it may even penalise organisations which have been able to make economies through efficiency gains'.[9] This is why our voluntary status is so important to maintain; we have discretionary funds that we use to put our patients' needs at the heart of our work and deliver new services as required. We are the breeding ground for innovation where new ideas are tested. Once new services have proven to be effective, they can be disseminated nationally into the smaller units in HSE hospitals. One of the positive initiatives to come from hospital groups, established in 2013, is the hub-and-spoke model which can be used to allow smaller units access to subspecialist services that they may not otherwise have been able to avail of. Consultants can travel maybe once a week to do a specialist clinic or provide a service in a small unit. I will discuss this further in Chapter 11.

7

LEADERSHIP IN PRACTICE

● ● ● ● ● ● ● ● ●

The mastership system is unique to the three Dublin maternity hospitals. It does not exist elsewhere in Ireland or the world. The Rotunda master is the chief executive officer and the clinical lead, and answers only to the hospital's Board of Governors. The executive management team is very small and, besides the master, includes only the director of midwifery and the secretary general manager, who looks after the administration and financial aspects of the hospital. This tight structure enables the executive to be responsive, innovative and supportive because reporting lines are very well laid out. The Board of Governors provides financial oversight, oversees appropriate indicators of performance and has the ability to drive changes and make decisions, including financial decisions. Every few years the board produces a strategy with an implementation plan and KPIs. They do that with the input of the executive team and key people within the hospital, but it is the board's own strategic plan and part of its responsibility.

This structure is similar to others in the voluntary sector, where the people who take responsibility for every aspect of a hospital's work actually understand the services. It is the reason why voluntary hospitals can undertake the sort of strategic thinking and strategic development that is lacking in HSE hospitals. If the people providing oversight are too remote from the hospital, they will not understand what is actually happening with the patients and the services on the ground. And the further away the governance is from the coalface, the greater the concentration on financial management rather than on clinical outcomes and quality of services, as is evident in HSE hospitals.

The Rotunda governance structure was devised by our founder, Bartholomew Mosse, and enshrined in the Royal Charter of 1756. The Coombe and Holles Street Hospital adopted the mastership system. The approach remains relevant and viable today despite recent suggestions that a complex modern hospital requires an equally complex organisational structure.[1] Voluntary hospital board oversight needs to be better recognised and acknowledged, and the model, perhaps, extended to HSE hospitals to allow them to improve the way they operate.

***

In the Royal Charter Bartholomew Mosse was very specific about the position of master in the Rotunda. The incumbent was to be the clinical lead for maternity and was to hold the position for seven years only. He – or now she – was to be appointed by the Board of Governors and was accountable to them. In the early days the hospital's service was confined to the labour ward and the antenatal ward, and the master understood everything that was happening. Today the activities of the hospital encompass the full range of medical and support services required by women and their newborn babies, maternity and gynaecology, neonatal and paediatrics, anaesthetics, radiology, assisted fertility, pregnancy prevention and termination, inpatients and outreach, as well as all of the auxiliary medical services such as pathology, medical social welfare and the supports. And still the master is in charge, taking the overview of every activity in the hospital, shaping the delivery of care and influencing the ethos of the hospital.

Today, with 270 beds and about 1,000 staff, the Rotunda Hospital is a busy and complex operation to run. Traditionally the master has been an obstetrician and gynaecologist, but as subspecialisation becomes more prevalent, it is likely that the person appointed to the role in the future will be a subspecialist, which will make oversight more difficult. Nevertheless, given that we are a single specialty hospital, whose role it is to improve outcomes for mothers and babies and provide a complete women's health service, with the right support it is still possible to be a clinical lead and hold the most senior administrative role.

Mosse's seven-year rule is a critical element in the design of the position; he wanted the master to be 'so bound up in the promotion of the hospital that … there was no time for his energies to become settled by custom and there was every incentive for him to work strenuously during the short term of his mastership'.[2] The seven-year term allows an opportunity to identify need and create change, to improve services, to ensure the changes bed down, and to audit how that change impacts and improves patient care. The cycle is so integral to the culture of the Rotunda that everyone working in the hospital expects change with the appointment of a new master. Change management can often be a difficult process, but when people expect a certain amount of change, introducing new services and procedures is made easier. There is also huge loyalty to the position of master within the hospital. This system or management structure encourages progress and innovation. It is a great way of making sure that the hospital remains up to date clinically and it generates a readiness to adapt quickly when change is needed.

Since our foundation we have had thirty-nine masters, each one an obstetrician or a gynaecologist, each approaching the post with their own visions, plans and ideas, and each bringing their own skills and attributes to the role. At various times in the life of the hospital different approaches, attitudes and initiatives were required to maintain the hospital at the forefront of care for women and babies. Sometimes it was financial control, at other times we needed to improve our research profile, and often we concentrated on improving and developing particular aspects of our clinical outcomes. In my case, I needed to reorganise the reporting relationships and structures to show evidence to the board and our funders that we were fully compliant, responsible and accountable in every aspect of our activities. I was also faced with a significant public relations role in order to maintain the hospital's reputation through some difficult and testing times as a whole series of negative stories about women's health emerged.

Until the 1980s the master was expected to live in the hospital with his family and be on call for twenty-four hours a day, seven days a week.[3] The original residence was in the east wing of the eighteenth-century hospital building and remained there for just over 200 years. In 1960, with the residence in a poor state of repair, the board converted it for hospital use and built a new house for the master within the grounds. George Henry, 1981–87, was the last master to live in. He had to be available for every issue that arose in the hospital, regardless of the time of day or night, and eventually his wife could take no more. According to legend she took his credit card and moved into the Shelbourne Hotel saying that she was not leaving there until he agreed to move out of the hospital, which he did. When Mike Darling was elected master in

1988, the Board removed the obligation that the master live on site. The home was converted for use for the hospital's HARI unit, created by Professor Robert Harrison.

For many years, the master was unpaid. He received a coal allowance but was expected to generate income through fees from pupils and assistants. This was to encourage him to promote and develop the teaching side of the Rotunda. The master could also build a very good private practice through his connection with the Rotunda, so financially this was a desirable position. A mid-nineteenth century suggestion of a fixed salary was dismissed by the Board of Governors, who were concerned that the master may become complacent, especially at a time when there was significant competition in Dublin for medical students.[4]

The administrative aspects of the job are formidable and masters have had to grapple with everything from budget and recruitment and training to infrastructure, the building, the utilities, overcrowding, allocation of space, temporary accommodation and new construction. Major new extensions such as the Thomas Plunket Cairnes Wing in 1895 and the new wing and entrance in 1993 took the efforts of several successive masters to achieve.

The master also makes key appointments. As the hospital expanded and medical science developed, masters would assess what direction they wanted a service to go in over the coming ten to fifteen years and make appointments accordingly. Even under the strict human resources guidelines of today, the master still has influence. If a new direction is required, or the master has a vision for a new service or development, a job description can be designed with a view to appointing someone with the relevant skills who can deliver on that vision. It is not a master's call as to who gets a job, but they can tailor the job description to reflect the direction in which they feel some aspect of the hospital's work should be going. Different masters have managed this process in different ways. In my case I took a collaborative approach and talked to key people to see what they thought before designing a new job description.

The ability to make important appointments is a key element in the independent nature of the voluntary hospital system and one we must fight to hold on to. The approach to appointments in the HSE hospitals is much more limited because hospital consultant appointments are made through the public administration system. Some of these hospitals do it better than others, but in many cases there is no representation from the hospital in question on the interview panels. It is hugely important to have a senior member of a team on a panel when interviewing for a consultant vacancy because it is critical that the new appointee fits in with the existing staff. If the hospital has no control over who they are going to get, problems can arise.

That said, it is difficult for HSE hospitals to attract consultants who have a great desire to make change. Creating change is so difficult and challenging that it needs the full and active support of management to achieve it. As was identified in the IRG report, HSE hospital management is too diffused, with parts of it so distant from the coalface that an ambitious person in that system is in danger of ending up as a generic consultant without the opportunity to get true value from their area of interest.[5]

***

The IRG report examined the governance of voluntary hospitals in detail and observed that their management boards are one of their key strengths.[6] This is definitely the experience of the Rotunda, where our Board of Governors scrutinises, constructively challenges and supports the master. In the early days the governors were actively engaged in fundraising and providing social support for the women and babies. The presence of influential and well-respected citizens would have encouraged others to support the work of the hospital. Today, corporate governance is more complex and requires board members to provide assistance to the executive, as well as making sure that the hospital management meets the required standards of accountability, integrity and propriety.

Our Royal Charter of 1756 provided for the establishment of a Board of Governors to provide non-executive direction to the hospital. The backgrounds of board members are varied but over the centuries all of them have worked and continue to work on a voluntary basis. Former masters are usually on the board. During my time, there were several very active members of the board, who were vocal and held sway. Some, including Gordon Linney, Hilary Prentice and Alan Ashe, served on multiple boards and had an in-depth knowledge of other voluntary hospitals in Dublin, which was very helpful at a time when the government approach to national healthcare management was changing fundamentally. For example, one of the issues Gordon Linney was acutely aware of was that of staying within budget. He wanted to make sure that the hospital finances were always very much in order and that we never got ourselves into debt because, he stressed to me, once the hospital gets into debt, the door is open for the HSE to come in and take over. Serious difficulties arise then, autonomy is eroded and it is very difficult to maintain independence in those circumstances. Another area that Gordon was alert to was that we were well ahead of the curve in terms of having women on the board: 'All through my time in the Rotunda we had a very strong female representation on the board and I think that was very important. In addition to their professional knowledge and skills set, they brought a softness and an understanding of the maternal to the board.'[7]

Our board takes a broad view, discussing topics that are or may become an issue for the hospital. Its purpose is to understand what is going on within the hospital, to oversee reports from the executive management team, and to strategically plan in what direction the hospital needs to go. The board is also essentially the ethics committee for the hospital. Issues like IVF, surrogacy and other sensitive matters are raised for discussion. And a subcommittee of the board signs off on the appropriateness of research and studies that are being run through the hospital.

With all of the national regulations relating to board members of every sort of organisation, people have a much greater understanding and awareness of what it means to be on a board now and the responsibilities involved. This makes it very important that voluntary board members especially are nurtured and looked after. We have been very lucky; the Rotunda board members are proactive in accessing formal support to deal with this. However, to continue with that governance model, the state should be investing in ways to support strong voluntary organisations, such as happens in Canada and other jurisdictions. Health is complex and very often the boards may not include enough people with expertise in health delivery, so they need help to ensure a really well-functioning voluntary board. At the moment in Ireland there are few available supports for boards, yet they are the lynchpin of the voluntary sector governance structure and their members all devote their time without charge.

***

The influence of the master in shaping the delivery of care cannot be understated. This role stretches right across every aspect of the hospital and includes the atmosphere and the ethos that permeates the everyday experience of staff and patients. Many former masters had an association with the hospital before taking up the position, so the Rotunda ethos was already imbued in them. They would have had an intimate working knowledge of the hospital and would have been known to staff, so, while their influence on the clinical and research work of the hospital was crucial, their influence on the atmosphere in the hospital was just as important. This influence is an aspect that I consider vital to our continued successful working relationships, good clinical outcomes and a good working environment.

The collegiate ethos has been supported in social as well as clinical ways, and there has been a terrific social life in the Rotunda for a long time. When the parties and other social events started is unclear, but Richard Dancer Purefoy, master from 1896 to 1903, was probably responsible for starting the popular tradition of carols at Christmas, which continued until the 1980s.[8] We also know that a fancy dress carnival in the early twentieth century led to a nurse being fired for lending her uniform to one of the postgraduate male doctors, who was seen wearing it while smoking and carousing with other doctors. In 1922, Gibbon Fitzgibbon, master from 1919 to 1926, began inviting resident students and nurses to the annual dance, which formerly had only been for a small, select group.[9] He had developed a strong, supportive relationship with his medical team during the War of Independence and the Civil War by using his influence to help the District team travel to and from the hospital during the curfew hours.

The social life for those working in the hospital in the 1940s was especially lively at Christmas time under the master Ninian Falkiner, who was aided by his wife and daughters. Falkiner was steering the hospital through the 'Emergency', the period of the Second World War, during which there was severe overcrowding as well as shortages in food and supplies. At the same time,.the staff were always on alert for emergency evacuation or for casualties in the event of an air raid. He brought in some well-known stars of the stage, such as Jimmy O'Dea, Noel Purcell and others, to provide impromptu entertainment in the large ward in the Thomas Plunket Cairnes Wing to raise the morale of the medical and nursing staff. Throughout the war, medical students knew that they could always get a hot shower in the students' mess in the Rotunda at any time of the day or night. After the war, the hospital attracted medical students and postgraduates, who were a cheerful bunch ready to party at any excuse. Falkiner was always invited and was more than happy to attend.[10]

The first master I met was Eric (Bill) Thompson, master from 1952 to 1959, but I was very young. My parents had been invited to his house in Sutton for a garden party and my abiding memory of that event was that he had an outdoor swimming pool and I spent the afternoon diving off the diving board. But I have no memory of him as a person.

Edwin Lillie, master from 1967 to 1973, was the first one that I would have known. He was a family friend and delivered me at home. I remember him from a very early age visiting the house. I would have known him as a consultant in the hospital when I was here as a medical student, but he had retired by the time I got my first job there. He was an incredibly kind, gentle sort of character and his kindness would be my overriding memory of him.

Ian Dalrymple, master from 1974 to 1980 was a different character. He had returned to his role as a consultant when I arrived as a junior and would have been more visible to me around the place. It was still too early in my career for me to comment on his clinical acumen or management, but he always had his finger on the pulse and knew exactly what was going on everywhere. He was a very dapper individual who always wore nice suits with a handkerchief in the breast pocket and kept his hair well oiled. He died in September 1996 and his funeral was held during the week I returned to the Rotunda.

George Henry, master from 1981 to 1987, was a larger-than-life character. People regarded him as a real west Brit, and he had the accent and the voice to go along with that. When he applied for the mastership and did not get it the first time around, he said he had to be master of something and went off to be master of the hunt. I was very fond of him. He was a very kind man with a strong social conscience and was all about caring for patients. He looked out for people who would have been less advantaged, and made sure that women had access to social workers. For example, rather than giving a patient directions to go down a corridor to see a social worker, he would take them there himself to make sure that they got everything that they were entitled to. George also pushed the envelope in terms of what was acceptable. He was one of the medical professionals who stood up to support the family planning clinic, which was radical at that time. He joined the board of the Fertility Guidance Company and persuaded the Rotunda to provide family planning services when they would not have been available in other places. In 1972, the Rotunda became the first Irish maternity hospital to set up a family planning clinic. It held two sessions a week and patients were prescribed the contraceptive pill, were given advice on the rhythm method or were referred to the Fertility Guidance Company if they wanted a diaphragm or IUD. Seven hundred and eight patients were seen in the Rotunda clinic that year.[11] George also made sterilisation available for those who needed it.

George was master when the Sexual Assault Treatment Unit (SATU) was opened in 1985. It was the first dedicated unit of its kind in Europe and has become a leader in providing medical and forensic treatment as well as supporting women and men over the age of fourteen who have experienced a sexual crime. Although traditionally a Rotunda consultant leads SATU and the service is situated on the hospital's grounds, it is an HSE service and is not under the governance of the Rotunda.

George was in charge of the hospital when funds were very tight. There was talk of reducing salaries and people not being paid for a week of work. At the same time the ceiling of the pillar room was in very bad repair, parts of it had fallen down, and it had to be fixed. So, while trying to provide services that were absolutely necessary for women in a modern obstetric service, he faced huge budgetary challenges.

I had a lot more to do with Michael Darling, who succeeded him in 1988. As master, Mike was very strict, with a stern, austere style. I remember being almost afraid of him when I was an SHO. That was the time when SHOs had to justify a particular intervention at perinatal and caesarean section meetings, and he could be intimidating. Mike and I had quite different personalities but once I got to know him, we got on very well. I worked very closely with him when I was a senior registrar and I found him very supportive and helpful. Obviously, I worked very hard for him and he paid that back in spades when it came to supporting me for consultant posts.

Outside work Mike was incredibly sociable, affable and a great party person, and he encouraged us to get involved in hospital parties and pantomimes. Each master has to have their own style and that depends on their personality type. Mike got the balance of work and play right, and showed me that there is a time and a place for a master to be firm and decisive because he or she is in charge and cannot be everybody's friend.

As well as being affable, Mike was very clever and very astute, and he used these characteristics to build a very good relationship with the Department of Health; we still had a line of communication there when he was master. Mike courted people in the department and got himself to the top table for the assistance and supplies that were required to run the hospital. At the end of his mastership, Mike made the following observation: 'Combining all the roles of management ultimately in one person, the master, has the great advantage of centralising and co-ordinating information, facilitating negotiations with the Department of Health and other bodies in securing the objectives of the hospital.'[12]

In the early 1990s some of the people I had trained and worked with moved to other hospitals but we maintained our links and came together to form a Ryder-Cup-style golf competition between the three hospitals. Within the Rotunda, anaesthetist Mary Bowen and myself formed a consultants' ski club. Each year around St Patrick's Day, we would go off to ski together for four days; Mike skied with us right through to the year before he died. It was from him that I picked up on the importance of generating social relationships among the staff. In particular, I learned from him that if you work together and play together, you do not annoy each other and you tend to help each other. We work in a very stressful hands-on job, where things can go very sour quickly and unexpectedly, and being able to call on your colleagues for support and help is vital. Supporting each other and working together are very much part of the job, and this is a very important message to teach younger colleagues. Therefore, instilling that sort of ethos and atmosphere throughout the Rotunda, in colleagues both senior and junior, is massively important.

One of Mike's more significant appointments was Ronan Gleeson, consultant in obstetrics and gynaecology. In the early 1990s, the management of gynaecological issues was changing and the master would have been looking out for someone who would bring new skills to the position. Until then there had been fewer treatment options for patients in their mid-to-late forties who were having difficulties with their periods. Hysterectomy was a common procedure at that time and when I started, we were probably doing two to four a day. Ronan Gleeson had trained in England and Australia and had returned with experience in endometrial and hysteroscopic resection of polyps and fibroids. His arrival probably marked the start of minimal access techniques in the Rotunda in place of open surgery, abdominal procedures and vaginal procedures. This initiated a new and hugely beneficial chapter of gynaecology surgery in the Rotunda, where the minimal access approach became more important. This then reduced the number of hysterectomies. Laparoscopy was also starting to become more common, but it was mostly diagnostic at that point. As time moved on, it became therapeutic and more procedures were done laparoscopically. Now we have minimal access surgery, endometrial resection, laser, endometrial ablation and the Mirena coil, and there are minimal access ways of managing those. The hysterectomy rate has gone way down over time and now we might only do two to three a week at most.

Mike Darling was a big advocate of tubal surgery and another major appointment during his mastership was Rishi Roopnarinesingh to bolster the fertility services. Rishi took over from Mike in surgical management of fertility issues.

Peter McKenna succeeded Mike in 1995 and continued to support the atmosphere of camaraderie without being quite so involved. Peter had been cross-appointed between the Rotunda and the Mater, and established our very important links with that hospital. As master, he used every opportunity to maintain and strengthen those links. Peter also developed good relationships with the Department of Health. He used to cycle quite a lot, and on the way to the department he would stop to buy a cake, then appear at a meeting in his cycling gear with a cake in hand.[13] Both Mike and Peter were excellent role models in how to develop important links outside the hospital with the organisations we required the assistance of from time to time.

***

In 2001, with Peter McKenna in the last year of his mastership, I applied for the post. I was also on the verge of being appointed a consultant. There is no doubt that when you become a consultant, you have a number of choices in terms of how you are going to make your mark. Some people do it through academia. Some people do it through their clinical presence and the service they provide. Some do it by developing a very substantial private practice. And some people are able to achieve the mastership and everything that goes with that. As I developed experience as an obstetrician and moved up the ladder, I was looking at what other people were doing and how they worked. I had worked for different masters and had seen their different styles, and over time I had decided that the mastership was something that I wanted. I had been brought up with the Rotunda. I had interacted with masters and consultants from the hospital who were friends with my parents from a very early age. I took summer jobs and had my obstetrics and gynaecology placement as a medical student here. It seemed like a natural progression. I felt I had something to give, that I owed the place something and it felt like the right thing to do. The Rotunda had given me a great amount and it felt that by going for the mastership I was giving back.

When considering applying for the mastership, there needs to be discussion at home, because it was not just about the applicant – the role involves one's whole family and has an impact on family life for a protracted period of time. The time has to be right in terms of children's ages, because over the course of seven years, children do a lot of growing up and a master is not going to be around the home quite as much. A master has to work very hard on being a master but also on their family relationships, because these can suffer; the job has taken its toll on the relationships of a number of Rotunda masters. Anyone applying for the position has to go into it with their eyes wide open and with family support. I thought long and hard about whether it was the right thing to do. Cathy, my wife, was fully supportive. She said to me that if I did not put my name forward, I would look back in fifteen or twenty years' time and regret that I never did. That was the key for me. It would be the pinnacle of my career. It would be an honour. It would be an achievement. Whether I got it or not was outside my control, but I felt that I needed to go for it, that it was a fulfilment of my destiny in many ways.

I was unsuccessful in 2001–2, but I had put myself forward and had prepared for the interview so I learned a lot more about the job. In retrospect I can see now that I would not have been ready for it. I was young and I had not worked as a consultant up to that point. It also gave me another seven years to prepare. I thought ahead and planned my strategy for the next time round.

The successful candidate and successor to Peter McKenna in 2002 was Mike Geary. Trained in Holles Street, Mike had rotated with me and had spent a year in the Rotunda as assistant master. On his return to Holles Street, he had applied for and got a fellowship training position in Toronto, but returned to Dublin on being appointed master of the Rotunda. A gregarious, affable character, he would have been very visible around the Rotunda during his year as an assistant master and was well known to the staff. That he was not yet a consultant was a little bit unusual, and it was the first time I was aware of, in recent times at least, that a non-consultant doctor was appointed as master in their first consultant role.

I got on very well with Mike. As colleagues we had a closer working relationship than I would have had with someone much older than me. Good communication is part of the master's job. Succession planning is also part of it and Mike was good at encouraging those who might be interested in going for the position next time around.

Several very important elements Mike brought to the role were his academic credentials and his interest in research. He also brought youth and enthusiasm, and a great interest in trainees. During his mastership he raised the research profile of the hospital to a new level with many more people going through the system doing MD and PhD theses and research projects. Subspecialist training was growing and to promote this he fostered links with Canada and the United States. He also made numerous appointments in the area of foetal medicine, including Fergal Malone, who was very well known and well respected worldwide in terms of his research output in the field. It was a massive coup to attract someone of his research experience and expertise. Raising the research agenda to a new level was undoubtedly one of Mike's biggest contributions as master.

***

The Dublin maternity hospital mastership system has been the subject of government interest, both positive and negative. In 2006, Judge Maureen Harding Clark praised the concept of the mastership in her report for the Department of Health and Children into the excessive use of peripartum hysterectomy at Our Lady of Lourdes Hospital in Drogheda. She pointed out how a mastership system would have benefited the Drogheda hospital:

> With no designated lead consultant [in the maternity unit of Our Lady of Lourdes Hospital] there was no system approaching the Mastership system, with its non-renewable tenure and the benefit of the introduction of new ideas to advance the practice of obstetrics and to improve the service offered to the public with each new Master. In the Dublin maternity hospitals it is the principal way in which a hospital can refurbish its ideas and keep itself up to date. This concept of changing leadership and renewal of ideas was sorely lacking in The Lourdes Maternity Hospital.[14]

Judge Clark noted that some of the midwives in the Drogheda hospital did not even know who was in charge. She stated that 'it was unlikely that any concerns within the Maternity Unit would be exchanged with the management of the general hospital, who were now seen as being driven by the North Eastern Health Board.'[15]

On the negative side, however, the mastership system has been questioned at official level on several occasions. When Mike Turner took up the seven-year mastership of the Coombe in 1992, he found out that there was a move to alter the position:

When I came into the post, the mastership in the Coombe was the weakest of the three hospitals and one of my tasks was to strengthen the role. The secretary manager was being replaced and the Department of Health had flagged to the chairman of our Board that they thought this was an opportunity to review the mastership of the hospital. They were keen to jettison it. However, we stood our ground, rewrote the general job descriptions of both the secretary manager and the director of midwifery. The board accepted that the master was chief executive and that the secretary manager reported to the master.[16]

Mike, who later was National Director, HSE Clinical Programme of Obstetrics and Gynaecology from 2010 to 2019, further observed to me:

The reason why the mastership system works so well is because we are competitive. We have seven years to innovate and bring in changes, and our entire focus and drive is directed towards that for that period. It is exhausting but it is what we sign up to do. The Department of Health and the HSE don't like the maternity hospital masterships because the masters go off and do things that they haven't approved of and they develop up new services and they are innovative and sometimes they might be a bit competitive but that competition is healthy in my view.

In 2007 the HSE commissioned the *Independent Review of Maternity and Gynaecology Services in the Greater Dublin Area* in which the mastership system was scrutinised. Undertaken by KPMG, the report was published in 2008. In the course of the review, the report

131

acknowledged, with regard to the mastership, that 'the clinical leadership and decision making [*sic*] has contributed to the hospitals' maintenance of acceptable performance levels within sub-standard facilities'.[17] The report also questioned its viability:

> From our stakeholder consultations it was clear that there was institutional loyalty to this system, but we question whether it is appropriate as a sustainable model for optimal clinical governance in a 21st century healthcare facility.
>
> We believe the system is out of step with most other healthcare institutions internationally and even within Ireland. The leader of the organisation is not only a practicing clinician but also the chief executive officer, which in today's climate of resource constraints, prudent budgetary management and necessary value for money, coupled with service evaluation and quality control, is an onerous workload which will prove impossible to manage in the future.[18]

The report suggested that the system should be replaced with a full-time chief executive officer and a clinical director for obstetrics and gynaecology.

A year after the KPMG report was published, I took over the mastership. With the governance structure being questioned and the HSE moving in on the voluntary hospitals, it was vital to use every opportunity to counteract those arguments and demonstrate the value of the mastership system and the importance of the voluntary system.

8

HEALTH CARE AND THE STATE

• • • • • • • • •

The modern Irish hospital network has diverse origins and successive governments have grappled with how to manage it as a whole – without quite succeeding. In the early years the state's role was to ensure that every county in Ireland had a reasonable hospital service. Now the state health authorities want to control the voluntary hospitals in the same way as they control their own former health board hospitals. In Dublin, as the city was expanding, the hospitals needed modernising and there was duplication of services among hospitals close to each other. Consequently, many of the voluntary hospitals that had been in existence for hundreds of years were transferred and absorbed into large teaching hospitals with boards appointed by the minister for health. These included Dr Steevens' Hospital, Sir Patrick Dun's and Mercer's, which were among those absorbed into St James's Hospital in the 1980s; Jervis Street and the Richmond, which were absorbed by Beaumont Hospital, opened in 1987; and the Meath, the Adelaide and the National Children's Hospital, which were all transferred to the new Tallaght Hospital in 1998. However, there are still about twenty-eight voluntary hospitals with their own legal governance, including some of the largest hospitals in Ireland.

Over the centuries the voluntary hospitals developed their own relationships with the government, before and after independence. From the beginning they raised their own funds, and in the mid-twentieth century, the voluntary hospitals organised the Irish Hospitals' Sweepstakes and were able to help the government hospitals with the money raised. Although the voluntary hospitals have also received an increasing amount of help from the government and today get the bulk of their funding from the state, they still raise a portion of their income themselves. Until the creation of the HSE by the 2004 Health Act, the voluntary hospitals communicated directly with the Department of Health and, in the case of the Rotunda, this worked very well. Issues were brought to the relevant people in the department for discussion and resolution. Major issues were taken to the secretary general or the minister of the department. It was a relationship of mutual respect and one that was never abused.

Since the early 2000s, there have been multiple changes in the way that health is organised in Ireland and several new layers of bureaucracy have been inserted between the Rotunda and government decision-makers. The HSE commenced in January 2005; in 2013 the government announced the creation of hospital groups, and in 2017 the reform proposal known as Sláintecare was launched. The HSE was given authority over the provision of all public health and social care services in Ireland, including the hospitals. Voluntary hospital funding from government was channelled through it, giving the HSE significant power over the distribution of funds. Numerous problems arose and the relationship became difficult. Since the hospital groups were set up – although in most cases not legally established – voluntary hospitals' access to the state health authorities has been through their own hospital group, which answers to the HSE, which in turn answers to the Department of Health. And all of the time voluntary hospitals like the Rotunda have their own legal and highly efficient governance authority, the autonomy of which is being squeezed by systems imposed by these multiple layers of government bureaucracy. The effect of this unwieldy bureaucratic system is to make communication, transparency and accountability much more difficult.

***

The Irish hospital system has its foundation partly in the voluntary hospitals of the eighteenth and nineteenth centuries, and partly in the network of infirmaries, dispensaries and hospitals of the nineteenth century funded by the government and ratepayers. The voluntary hospitals were mostly based in the cities and provided health services to the poor and destitute. The government and local authority services, especially those in rural Ireland, were often of very poor quality and only the indigent used them, as people with means visited a doctor privately.

In 1838 the Irish Poor Law Act led to the network of 163 workhouses constructed in Ireland over the following thirteen years. Each workhouse was to be funded by local rates and was to include an infirmary. However, the construction coincided with the Great Famine and the workhouses became infamous places where the destitute went as a last resort. From the 1860s onwards, the situation in workhouses improved; the government paid for medication and for half of the salary of the medical officers, and religious sisters nursed the sick. Although conditions were still basic, it was somewhere that poor sick people could go. By the end of the century at least one-third of those in workhouses were clinical patients. The facilities varied in quality from well-equipped surgical hospitals by the standards of the day to those that were barely distinguishable from the original workhouse infirmary. In 1898 the Local Government (Ireland) Act transferred control of the workhouses to newly formed county councils, but the quality of the health care remained patchy. Meanwhile the voluntary hospitals, although struggling to maintain service on limited resources, continued to develop their clinical practices under the authority of their boards. Many, like the Rotunda, were incorporating the latest medical research into their work.

In 1919 the Irish Public Health Council was appointed, recognising that the government had a duty to provide health care not only to the destitute but to everyone who needed it. The council's ambition was to bring hospital services together under a strong central health authority, but it was faced with the challenge of persuading all the local authorities to cooperate. In the meantime, the council increased financial assistance for the voluntary hospitals, some of which were in danger of closing if help was not forthcoming. Following independence in 1922, the concept of the workhouse ended, but the medical services – the hospitals, the infirmaries and the dispensaries – continued on, now under the control of the minister for local government and public health. The 1947 Health Act established the Department of Health, which took over responsibility for all health services, including hospitals. In 1953, the act extended access to hospital care with little or no charge to over 80 per cent of the population. Four years later, the Voluntary Health Insurance (VHI) was established for those who were above the threshold and could afford private insurance. Meanwhile private nursing homes were providing maternity services for women who could afford it and who, in the past, would probably have given birth at home.

In 1968, a report into the Irish hospital sector commissioned by the minister for health recommended a considerable reduction in the number of hospitals providing acute services and a concentration of services into a smaller number of larger hospitals.[1] The report, known as the Fitzgerald Report, also stressed the need for closer coordination of the voluntary and public hospital systems. The report led to the establishment of Comhairle na nOspidéal, a statutory body established under the Health Act of 1970 that advised the minister on matters relating to the organisation and operation of hospital services, and regulated the number and type of consultant posts. The same act created eight regional health boards. In 1999, one of these, the Eastern Health Board, which incorporated Counties Dublin, Wicklow and Kildare, was split into three regional health boards and one regional authority, giving a total of eleven health authorities in the twenty-six counties. The Fitzgerald Report had made recommendations concerning maternity services around Ireland, and by 1989 most of the smaller maternity units had closed and the great majority of births were taking place in a hospital or unit in which the annual number of births exceeded 1,500. Better facilities led to better outcomes and infant mortality rates dropped.[2]

Recent government initiatives to manage the hospital network began in the early 2000s, when Minister for Health Micheál Martin proposed a new health act, which was passed in 2004 after Mary Harney took up the ministry. Comhairle na nOspidéal and the eleven regional health authorities were dissolved and their functions transferred to the HSE, which came into being in January 2005. The voluntary hospitals and other voluntary health services were identified in the act under two sections, 38 and 39, and they were to receive their government funding through this new executive. Thirty-five voluntary bodies were classified as Section 38 organisations; of these, seventeen received between €40 million and €250 million in 2017.[3] They included St Vincent's Hospital, the Mater, Mercy Hospital Cork and St John's Hospital Limerick, as well as the Rotunda and the other two Dublin maternity hospitals. All the staff in the Section 38 hospitals were now classified as public servants and became subject to the standard salary scales for the health sector, as well as having access, in the main, to a public service pension scheme. Section 39 is a much larger cohort, with agencies of all sizes, and includes hospices, disability services, mental health providers, nursing homes and homecare providers, as well as small community-based groups and social care services.

The Rotunda, as a Section 38 hospital, now had restrictions on making new appointments, which curtailed our independence to some degree. While we retained some autonomy over replacement appointments, any new position had to be approved by the HSE because all new appointments came with long-term costs, including the pension commitments associated with public service positions. There may also have been other cost implications, such as administrative back-up or facilities needed to run a particular service, so we now had to make a case to the HSE to support new positions. However, if the hospital could develop a service with existing staff and no headcount implications, we could carry on as before and it was not an issue. So now, unlike the statutory hospitals, we can hire people without reference to the HSE and give them a Rotunda contract so long as we stay within a stipulated headcount.

**

The Health Act 2004 and the establishment of the HSE made a fundamental difference to the Rotunda's relationship with the government agencies. Before that, we had had a very good working relationship with the Department of Health. When there were issues and concerns, the master could get to the top table. Peter McKenna recalled:

It was all very simple then, the hospital had a relationship with the Department of Health. I knew a whole raft of people down there and brought different problems to different people, depending on who was geared to sort them out. You didn't go bothering them unless you had a significant problem but if you did, you went and you got a fair hearing. And if they had a problem, they would contact the hospital directly. It was all very straightforward. I didn't have to deal with the health boards or their hospitals. The health boards looked after the community side of things and did not have any relationship with the voluntary hospitals.

Then, the former staff of the health boards became the HSE and two groups that had never worked together before needed to establish a relationship. Our personal connections with individuals in the Department of Health were gone, as the HSE became the intermediary between the hospital and our source of funding. However, the staff of the HSE had had little or no interaction with the voluntary hospitals before this and did not seem to understand us. Difficulties arose and the relationship gradually turned sour to the point it arrived at in 2019 when the IRG report described it as 'fractured'.

In retrospect it is possible that the lack of understanding on the part of both the new HSE and the voluntary hospitals contributed to a tense relationship from the beginning. The voluntary boards and their senior executives may not have understood the new executive or what was needed for us to fit into the new structure. We were so used to our independence and doing things our own way that we probably dug our heels in and questioned the need to report to this new body and to produce data in different formats just to suit it. The HSE, on the other hand, was born out of the health boards and was so used to controlling its own hospitals that it may not have understood that the governance of the voluntary hospitals was different. The HSE style was very managerial and very financially orientated, and it did not really get where we were coming from and did not seem to understand the value that the voluntary sector brings to the health service. Looking back, the voluntaries should have talked to the HSE more during this early period and explained our governance structure. By presuming that they understood us, we probably missed an opportunity to engage them with the benefits of the voluntary model. The failure on both sides to communicate and to understand where the other side was coming from has contributed to the poor relationship between the two.

During my mastership, I believe that the HSE officials that I dealt with found the voluntary hospital model difficult. To them the key metric in hospital management was all about control and managing a budget, and they had no interest in clinical outcomes. Our KPIs were clinical as well as financial, and in order to deliver a quality service, we had to manage risk, but this was not appreciated or understood by the management of the HSE at the time. We had to collect information, which was then passed up through the hierarchy in the HSE to their senior executive team, who were, in turn, answerable to the minister for health and the Department for Finance. The message coming back to the HSE from the Department of Finance was probably all about controlling spending, so that would have filtered through every level of their organisation and set the agenda for the HSE officials.

The differences in emphasis led to huge frustration on our part and made dealing with the HSE extremely challenging. I was looking at clinical data, dealing with crises and potentially tragic situations, while the officials in the HSE were only interested in budget and headcounts. We were not being treated as trusted partners and there was no credit given to the fact that our job was to manage clinical risk as well as our finances; that our board has a duty to manage finances and be responsible in the way we manage our budget got lost in the conversation. By the HSE refusing to engage with the health of patients, it was difficult to get any sense of partnership with the body that was supplying much of our funding. It was only really when something became a political issue, like patients on trolleys or the Covid pandemic, that the HSE would change its focus, and this was incredibly frustrating for us.

The link between the voluntary hospitals and the HSE shifted in 2013 when the hospital groups became the intermediary between the two. Although the hospital groups other than the Children's Hospital Group do not have any legal status, a Section 38 voluntary hospital's funding comes through its respective group. This will be discussed in a later chapter.

***

The HSE's relationship with the voluntary hospitals is based on the fact that it is the channel through which we received our state funding. During my professional lifetime, the Rotunda received around 80 per cent of its income from the government, which pays for the salaries and the day-to-day running of the hospital. As a Section 38 hospital, there is also an expectation and an onus on us to bring in our own money, which we do through various means, such as accommodation fees from private and semi-private patients. We have discretion as to how we use the funds we raise ourselves; we also have discretion as to how we use the money provided by the government subject to an annual SLA and the obligation to remain within the stipulated headcount.

As a voluntary hospital, fundraising efforts have been essential to support the work of the Rotunda to a greater or lesser extent since the beginning. The hospital was founded as a charity and at first its source of income was entirely through fundraising, philanthropy and benevolence. Bartholomew Mosse incorporated features into the plan for the hospital to support the hospital's fundraising activities. In 1803 the Rotunda successfully petitioned parliament for a grant to augment the funds of the hospital.[4] This became a regular grant, but, crucially, the Rotunda ran its affairs independently of any public relief scheme.

As time went on, the hospital became more dependent on municipal and government funds and patient contributions. In 1919 the master, Gibbon Fitzgibbon, was a man who exercised a rigid economy. The hospital had debts when he took over and, amongst other things, he organised a very successful bazaar in Ballsbridge to raise funds. Nevertheless, he had to close the pathological laboratory and he could not afford to install an X-ray department.[5] So from the 1920s the hospital was forced to switch to a policy of charging patients something to put towards paying for the various services. By 1933 three mothers in four paid something towards their care.[6]

Following independence in 1922 and the ensuing hard economic times, health services were low on the priority list. Desperate to upgrade and improve services in line with developments in medical science and patient care, Holles Street Hospital, together with five other voluntary hospitals, organised the first Irish Hospitals' Sweepstakes. The government supported the move with the necessary legislation and the Sweepstakes became very successful. Six sweepstakes raised £2.7 million. The Rotunda's Board of Governors was reluctant to participate, but the amounts of money being raised were significant and the board was persuaded to join in on the fifth sweepstake in 1933.[7]

The Hospitals' Sweepstakes was promoted internationally and over its fifty-seven-year history, it brought substantial amounts of money into the country, especially from the United States. While the lottery had been set up by the voluntary hospitals for their own benefit, a series of acts in 1931–33 gave the minister for local government and public health control over the sweepstakes and allowed the bounty to be shared with local government hospitals. In the Rotunda, the master was able to carry out improvements, including a new nurses' home and a large outpatient clinic.[8]

Our dedicated fundraising arm, incorporated in 1973 as Friends of the Rotunda and later renamed The Rotunda Foundation, is a charity independent of the hospital and state, but all of its efforts are for the hospital and its work. It now manages the renovated Pillar Room complex, the Hospital Shop and the car park, and leases the Gate Theatre and the old Ambassador cinema. It continues to be very active and fundraises for research and for specialist pieces of equipment, but it does not fund the running of the hospital or salaries.

We also raise income through fees for private and semi-private patients, donations and bequests. The role of discretionary income is a very important aspect of the voluntary hospital system. The IRG report noted that voluntary organisations have contributed large sums of money over the years to the building of new facilities, purchase of new equipment, and the provision of financial support for staff training and research activities.[9]

***

In the late 1990s, a hospitals' accreditation system was introduced in Ireland. It covered all aspects of a hospital, not just clinical work. In order to meet accreditation standards, each hospital had to have written evidence to demonstrate that it had guidelines and systems in place. It was a step in the process of going towards uniformity of health services in Ireland. Before I was appointed consultant in 2002, I was given time by Peter McKenna to train as an accreditation assessor. It was a big administrative and bureaucratic exercise in terms of managing all our procedures, protocols and guidelines, and gathering all the written evidence required to show how we did things. We embraced it because it was the modernisation of the way we thought and the way we worked. The Rotunda was the first maternity hospital to achieve this accreditation, so, in that way, it set the standard. It was a lot of work and bureaucracy and, consequently, many people regarded it as a waste of time. But it formalised our way of doing things and anyone from the outside looking in could see that we were a forward-thinking institution confident about focusing on how we could improve any aspect of our work.

This accreditation process lasted for only a few years before it was taken over by the Health Information and Quality Authority (HIQA), which was established under the 2007 Health Act. HIQA, as part of its brief to monitor the safety and quality of Irish healthcare, comes into the hospital and looks in detail at how we manage a particular area. The work we had done as part of the accreditation assessment had tidied up our paperwork; we had systems and protocols and guidelines in place that we could adapt to satisfy HIQA standards, so it made it a lot easier for us. This commitment to improving processes is a key part of what enables us to be both self-determining and accountable at the same time.

As the government continued to look for ways of streamlining the Irish hospital network, Minister for Health Mary Harney believed that co-location was the way forward. The conversation about relocating the Dublin maternity hospitals started in 2007, with the KPMG review into maternity and gynaecology services in Dublin. Their report, published in 2008, looked at various different options and suggested that the Rotunda should co-locate with the Mater Hospital, that Holles Street should co-locate with St Vincent's Hospital, and that the Coombe should co-locate with either St James's Hospital or Tallaght Hospital. The conversation about the ultimate fate of the existing Dublin maternity hospitals had started.

At the time of writing, there have been all sorts of bumps along the way. Arising out of Minister James O'Reilly's hospital group proposal of 2013, the Rotunda is now expected to co-locate with Connolly Hospital in Blanchardstown. Interestingly this co-location was dismissed in the KPMG report. In British terms, Connolly Hospital would be a district general hospital rather than a major acute general hospital, and it was not regarded as strong enough in terms of its facilities and specialities to be the co-location partner of the Rotunda, which is a national referral unit for sick mothers and babies. This issue still hangs in the air and will be discussed further in Chapter 11.

9

THE MASTERSHIP: LEARNING TO MANAGE RISK

● ● ● ● ● ● ● ● ●

O n 1 January 2009 I took up the mastership of the Rotunda. The position had been advertised in late 2007 by which stage there would have been plenty of speculation about who would be applying for it. The announcement that I had been successful was made in early summer 2008, which gave the staff six months to get used to the idea and gave me time to prepare myself. My vision was to make the Rotunda Hospital *primus inter pares*, first among equals, and for it to be the preeminent maternity hospital in the country in every way it possibly could. I had identified areas that I wanted to address, which would not necessarily turn the place upside down but would build on the good work that was already being done and move the hospital forward from a reputational point of view.

When I took over the job, the country had already entered a period of recession and a huge crisis in public finances. At the same time, we experienced a massive increase in the numbers of patients coming to the hospital due to the arrival of many young people from the European Union during the Celtic Tiger years. We were also managing more high-risk patients with complex comorbidities and diverse medical and social issues. Statistically we delivered more patients per annum over those seven years than we did in any other seven years in the history of the hospital. And we were doing this while being squeezed on budget and staff numbers.

I was lucky I had a strong team. Pauline Treanor, ex-director of midwifery, was the hospital secretary general manager, Margaret Philbin was the new director of midwifery, and there was a strong and supportive Board of Governors. But we were now in an era where the buzz words were governance and accountability. The practice of organ retention, which became a national issue just as I took over, would show us that our reporting systems were not as good as they should have been and needed to improve. Our governance and the oversight of our increasingly diverse services also had to improve and be seen to have improved. With so much activity in the hospital, it was more difficult for one person – the master – to oversee all areas directly, so reporting, middle management and committee structures needed to be revamped. Together with my management team, this was one of my first tasks and I think it would have been much more difficult to achieve in any other type of hospital. But the Rotunda staff expected change and they all had the desire to repair any reputational damage to the hospital arising from the practice of organ retention. This made leading that change much easier.

A big issue that interested me was the question of leadership within the hospital. We had good leadership at every senior level, but I felt that the lower and middle levels of management within the hospital could do more by showing more initiative and taking a bit more ownership of issues relevant to them. I was aware that the culture before my mastership was very much 'the master is in charge, the master will decide'. But this was changing too, especially as there were people around the table who knew a lot more about the subject in question than the master did. I took a view that my mastership was going to be more like a prime minister with a cabinet of people advising on their area of expertise rather than me making unilateral decisions.

As master it was up to me how much clinical work I would do alongside the administrative work. I chose a balance of about 20 to 30 per cent clinical and 80 to 70 per cent administrative. Being in a position to maintain a hands-on role is the beauty of the job. Not everyone chooses to do that; for example Sharon Sheehan, master of the Coombe from 2013 to 2019, did 100 per cent administration. But for me, doing a percentage of clinical work at the coalface kept me current; and from a staff morale point of view, it was good to know that the master was going to be on the labour ward, in the clinic, or in theatre. Being easily accessible was tricky at times, but, overall, it was useful.

However, before I did anything, I had to deal with the massive issue of organ retention. I knew it was coming down the line, as did the board. It was to be my first task and a very high-profile one. It was at a time when people were demanding national institutions to be accountable and responsible, and it was critical that as a hospital we managed it well.

***

The issue of organ retention in hospitals had been bubbling under the surface for some time. In 1998 it had emerged in Britain that it was a practice in some hospitals to retain the organs of stillborn babies or those who had died just after birth so that autopsies and research could be carried out. Over the following ten years cases of this having happened in Ireland emerged and questions were asked. There was significant turmoil around it. The Rotunda was at the centre of the story. Patient care is our priority, but a considerable amount of research is also undertaken. Since the earliest days, the Rotunda has researched the causes of maternal and infant deaths in order to learn from them. Gathering information is a core activity in a maternity hospital and our dedicated obstetric pathology service has a track record of being able to establish the cause of death accurately for women and their families because we painstakingly look at every possibility for the cause behind every neonatal death and stillbirth. Today our pathology department is a network of laboratories separated by subspecialisations including microbiology, biochemistry, haematology and histopathology, each with a team of senior scientists and consultants.

In the case of a stillbirth or a death just after birth, the pathologist's job is to find out why this happened. In order to do this, they need to gather information and pull it together into a report. It takes time to assemble what is required. Processes need to be followed and these are complex, so it can take weeks to create accurate post-mortem reports. In Ireland, culturally, the time from death to burial is very quick, so, as in other hospitals, the pathology department in the Rotunda had retained many tissue samples. In some instances, whole organs had not been returned to the baby before burial. At the time and historically it was considered too much for a bereaved couple to have to deal with being told that we were retaining their baby's organs for a post-mortem. This was an outdated and paternalistic approach, and when it emerged that this had been happening, people were, rightly, very unhappy about it. As obstetricians, we did not fully understand the laboratory's processes and when we found out about it, obviously something had to be done.

The Rotunda was subject to much of the publicity around this practice. As master it was my job to accept responsibility on behalf of the hospital for the practice. I was transparent in identifying what had happened. It was hugely difficult and traumatic for the hospital, and an equally difficult time for the parents. We realised that parents and families who had lost babies were now going to hear about this for the first time, so we set up a helpline in preparation for the response. We also knew that the publicity generated by this issue would reignite trauma for women who may have had a post-mortem done on their baby. As it happened, women who had had difficult, traumatic deliveries up to fifty years earlier came forward and we dealt with those cases even if they had not been affected by organ retention.

We met all of the affected families and we moved quickly to change the process. Now organs are sampled and returned to the body before burial. If there is an unusual situation where the organ has to be retained, we talk to the couple and explain the case. In the past, people used to give verbal consent to a post-mortem. A lot of people did not even remember that a post-mortem had been done because they were so traumatised. It is now very much an open transparent process that is fully consented in writing, with copies of the consent being given to the parents.

Partly arising from this, our bereavement services were transformed, as we recognised that bereavement was an area that needed to be invested in with improved facilities and staffing. The Rotunda had had bereavement services through our social workers who were assigned to the neonatal unit and to the paediatric team. They helped with the stress and grief of those who had been bereaved, or those who had to accept the burden of an infant suffering from a physical or neurological injury. Since the 1970s, there had been new thinking around management of bereavement through miscarriage, stillbirth, neonatal death and sudden infant death syndrome.[1] At the time the state did not register stillbirths, but the Rotunda tried to overcome this by giving parents a certificate of stillbirth to acknowledge its reality. In 1980 the old mortuary in the Rotunda, a stark forbidding place, was redesigned and replaced by a smaller mortuary with a waiting room. A beautifully lined Moses basket was provided by Dr Stella MacClancy of the Samaritan Fund Committee. The committee also provided a camera for photographs, a memory box to hold the photos, an identity bracelet, details of weight, a lock of hair if possible, a footprint, the autopsy report, and the birth and death certificates. It all helped. In 1984 the Irish Stillbirth and Neonatal Death Society, founded by a group of bereaved parents, issued a useful booklet entitled *A Little Lifetime*. The master, the matron and the head medical social worker of the Rotunda were consulted in its preparation. The society also formulated a memorial service for babies who died before or shortly after birth. In the early 1990s, the medical social workers provided therapeutic counselling for bereaved parents on an individual or a group basis. Registration of stillbirths became a legal requirement in 1994.

Arising from the organ retention issue we recognised that there was now also a need for clinical back-up and dedicated midwifery in this area. Success in dealing with an adverse outcome lies with communication, help from specialist staff, perinatal pathology and open disclosure. We embraced this approach completely. There are always situations that are difficult to deal with, but, in the majority of those, patients are grateful for an open and honest approach. We realised that it was not enough to have just one person in the bereavement services who, when unavailable, had no one covering for them. We needed succession planning and more people coming on stream to assist. Any type of pregnancy loss, no matter what stage of pregnancy it happens at, is emotive and a big life event for the parents, and we wanted to ensure that we were able to provide the best possible assistance. So, during my mastership, we wrote a new set of guidelines in relation to bereavement care and the management of bereaved mothers, and we streamlined the service to improve it and ensure that nothing was missed.

***

In broader terms the organ retention issue had raised a red flag in terms of management oversight in all areas of the hospital. There was a gap in the clinical governance structure and everyone in the hospital recognised this. It was something I now had to address and at the same time it gave me an opportunity to stamp my authority on the hospital. Over a relatively short space of time, we had gone from the situation where the master had understood everything in the hospital because it was all obstetrics and gynaecology, to a situation where the breadth of our services was much greater and it was impossible for the master to know and understand what was happening in every corner. We had much bigger departments and multiple clinics, and lots of people working in the hospital who had a degree of expertise and an oversight of their piece of the service, which the master could not fully understand. The reporting structure had not evolved to take that into account. With the help of Pauline Treanor and Margaret Philbin, we put a huge amount of effort into addressing management at every level and overhauling the committee reporting structure.

The new system of reporting had to reassure the master that everything going on within the hospital was working appropriately and that everyone was meeting the relevant standards and quality in every aspect of their work. We introduced performance management to the entire hospital. KPIs were devised and agreed upon with each department. Each area reported specifically on their KPIs, which were then brought to the executive management team and on to the board. In this way the master could formally assure the board that every department was on top of their KPIs. Specialists were asked to make recommendations in their field, present me with evidence, demonstrate that this was the right thing to do, and then we would go ahead and do it. I was not in a position to overrule them on their recommendations, and this is where changing the committee structure and giving people accountability came in. The master cannot have eyes on absolutely everything, but they have executive responsibility and are ultimately responsible for what is going on, so they have to trust their system of reporting and good management.

The Rotunda Board of Governors realised that they also needed to take responsibility for the oversight of the growing number of departments in a more structured manner. This was a time nationally when boards of all organisations were being encouraged to be accountable in a more formal way. It was no longer appropriate for the chair of our board to ask the master at a board meeting whether everything was okay and then accept the assurance that yes, there was no need to worry. This is an oversimplification of the situation but roughly speaking it was a bit like that. The board would have been very trusting of the master and the executive management team, and would have accepted assurances that all was well. Alan Ashe, Hilary Prentice and Patricia Walsh were the three chairs of the board during my mastership. All were extremely supportive and caring, just as one would expect. They gave appropriate levels of oversight, were interested in seeing how things were improving, put pressure on to ensure that everything was done correctly and checked that there was the appropriate level of reporting.

Each month I produced a written report for the board with KPIs in the different areas, and escalated issues and concerns arising. Then, if it was perceived that there was a need for closer scrutiny on anything, the issues were discussed. For example, over the course of six months the board monitored the KPIs in pathology and the post-mortem service on a monthly basis to see that everything was being done in a timely manner and there was no indication of organs being retained. When they were happy that we had a system in place and it was working, they left it up to the master to keep an eye on those areas and the level of board oversight dropped back. This evolution happened quite quickly and within two years we had gone from verbal reassurances from the master to the board, to structured board meetings with focused and rigid examination of the KPIs. Put together with hospital accreditation, HIQA and other government overseeing agencies monitoring our standards, it was a big cultural shift for the Rotunda. We were now firmly in an era of complete transparency and accountability across the whole organisation.

Meanwhile the board maintained its role in providing oversight on sensitive issues as they arose. For example, aspects of assisted fertility were matters of concern as the relevant science and technology moved ahead of the law. During my mastership several national issues were discussed at board level, including the death of Savita Halappanavar, Professor Oonagh Walsh's *Report into Symphysiotomy in Ireland, 1944–1984*, and the reports of infant deaths and adverse events in the maternity unit in the Midlands Regional Hospital in Portlaoise. Issues concerning women's health were being raised in the media, and each time that happened there would have been a report at board level to reassure the governors that the Rotunda was not exposed in relation to the particular issue.

***

With 62,423 babies born in the Rotunda during my mastership, this was the busiest seven-year period in terms of obstetric activity in the history of the hospital and it coincided with a severe recession. The population of the city had increased, there were more people of childbearing age and there was a massive boom in the number of babies being delivered. When I started as a senior house officer, the Rotunda would have been seeing around 8,300 patients a year with 5,000–6,000 deliveries. During my mastership there were on average around 10,000 patients per year during those seven years – including miscarriages and ectopic pregnancies – and in 2014 it peaked at nearly 10,967.[2] The Coombe and Holles Street were equally busy, but the numbers in the rest of the country had dropped. This was because the Rotunda serves north Dublin, the Fingal area and parts of Meath, an area where many young couples live. We also had people coming to the Rotunda from Wicklow, Kildare and Wexford, often bypassing other hospitals. Of course, at the same time people from Howth or Sutton would sometimes bypass us and go to Holles Street or the Coombe – people have different reasons for choosing a specific maternity hospital.

For some years prior to the recession, roughly 20 to 30 per cent of our patients had been private or semi-private and we had relied on their accommodation fees to plug the funding gap. However, during the recession many people did not renew, or did not take out, or chose not to use their private insurance, and the numbers of private and semi-private patients attending the hospital dropped off by 30 per cent. Those patients were still coming to the hospital, so we were getting more activity but less funding, both from the state and from private sources – it was a double hit.

As our obstetric activity dramatically increased, postnatal accommodation became an issue and we had to reduce the length of stay. We discharged women who had had a normal delivery after one day rather than the more usual three days. We reduced the stay following a caesarean section from five days to three. At the same time, we improved our community services so a team of midwives would call to the patients at home to make sure that everything was satisfactory. In some cases, however, we held on to the patient and used Jurys Hotel in Parnell Street as a spillover for antenatal and postnatal care. It was all about finding solutions that were within our control. We also had extra beds placed in the big Nightingale wards with curtains in-between each patient, which was not ideal as the beds were pretty close together and this also gave us major infrastructural issues around showers and toilets in the older part of the hospital, with lots of patients sharing one or two toilets or one or two baths. We were not in compliance with HIQA standards, yet we received no infrastructural investment from the HSE to help to make us compliant.

In relation to staffing, we were restricted in making new appointments because we were now a Section 38 hospital under the 2004 Health Act. The main response I could make in those circumstances was to ensure that we had enough junior staff to keep the place safe and to reduce stress levels for everybody. We went from one registrar on call at night to having two available so we could deal with situations as they arose. It became a two-tier system with a senior and a junior registrar on call at all times.

We did think very carefully about capping the numbers of patients that we booked in – we talked about it and threatened it, but, ultimately, we decided that it was not a safe thing to do. If they remained unbooked, it meant that no one was looking after them. There are certain things that need to happen at different stages of pregnancy, including the initial risk assessment, anatomy scans and dating of pregnancy, and if those things are not done at the appropriate time, there is an associated clinical risk. Our approach was the lesser of two evils – there was a clinical risk involved in rising levels of activity, but there was also a clinical risk in having people unbooked.

The other side of this high level of activity was that our maternity and gynaecology services were competing with each other on the same site. The rising intervention and caesarean section rates took up extra time in theatres and that reduced our capacity for gynaecology procedures. This was a situation with serious implications for women. In the hospital system generally, the major acute hospitals concentrated on gynae oncology, while the general hospitals manage benign gynaecology services. But the general hospitals were under such pressure, they did not have the theatres, the staff, the beds or the facilities to look after elective patients, so they reduced their levels of benign gynaecology services. At the Rotunda we are very aware of how many gynaecological issues affect women's everyday lives. Someone, for example, who is having significant menstrual issues can be in distress for one or two weeks out of every four, and this can have an enormous impact on their lives, their families and their work. Also, it is important to note that all gynaecology starts off as benign. A patient usually does not get a diagnosis of gynaecology cancer until they have been through the routine screening services and have been triaged upwards.

For north Dublin, the Rotunda is the principal provider of benign gynaecology services. The Mater deals exclusively with gynae oncology, and the gynaecology units in Beaumont and Connolly are small. A private patient had the option to go to the Mater or the Bon Secours Hospital, but public gynaecology patients in north Dublin in the early years of my mastership struggled to get into a hospital for an elective procedure, and even if they could get into one of the other hospitals, those elective gynaecology lists were cancelled as soon as there was a trolley crisis. This eventually became a political issue.

During all of this time the challenge of managing the activity and risk within the hospital was difficult, but I felt that we got little or no help from the HSE in relation to any of these matters. At the beginning of my mastership I was of the view that if we had a major problem at a hospital with the numbers going up and the situation becoming unsafe, then the state health authorities would do their best to try and help us to reduce the risk. I believed that there was a strong possibility that someone might listen if I went to them and explained the risk. But that was not the reality. In retrospect I can now see that we were working with different metrics – ours were clinical while theirs were budgetary. At the time, however, I was only concerned about managing the hospital through a period of severe pressure.

In 2012 we had 10,397 deliveries, the highest annual activity level to that point in the history of the hospital. There were times where we had multiple emergencies one after the other, or even at the same time, putting a huge strain on our staff and resources. I was really concerned that the place had become dangerously busy. As master I went to the HSE to raise the issues. I was coming from an institution where if we have a problem, we work together and do something to resolve it. However, when I presented my concerns to senior people within the

HSE and stressed how serious the situation was, one official made it very clear to me: 'It is your risk, you manage it.'

I was shocked, it was not what I was expecting and found it really frustrating and annoying. It would have been much more productive if the HSE had acknowledged that we had issues in relation to overcrowding and infection control concerns. It would also have been helpful if they had accepted that postnatal women were being looked after in facilities that were not fit for purpose anymore, and then offered to work in partnership with us to find a constructive solution. When I thought about it afterwards, what this official meant was that if our labour wards were too busy, then it was up to us to turn off some element of our activity, close the theatres, stop doing gynaecology and divert our resources to the labour ward. We had already curtailed our gynaecology lists, which meant that the waiting list to see outpatients was getting out of control. The Rotunda Board of Governors, recognising the clinical risk, agreed to fund a waiting list initiative and pay for patients, especially those at risk of a cancer diagnosis, to be operated on in the Mater Private.

When I did not get any traction in the HSE, I escalated my concerns to the Department of Health and the minister. Minister for Health James Reilly did hear about it, but his attitude was that we were going to be co-located with Connolly Hospital in Blanchardstown as part of his 2013 hospital group scheme and everything would be okay then. But that move was so far in the future that this response did not bring any immediate relief to our circumstances. I met Minister Reilly on a couple of occasions and I came away from those meetings deflated, thinking that our concerns about high activity levels and clinical risk were not being taken seriously.

My communications with the HSE continued to be unsatisfactory. In years gone by, when the master would have dealt with a small number of officials in the Department of Health, those officials recognised that the Rotunda provided an important function, relationships were developed and with that came trust and understanding on both sides. But during my mastership, there was no one person within the HSE with whom I, as head of a hospital, could speak and have these sorts of discussions. Those assigned to that role moved out of the job so quickly that I ended up working with a succession of five different people.

Communication and good relationships with our funders and with the people who run the health service are critical elements in the development of a quality service. With the rapid changes in personnel, I could not build up a relationship with any one person in the HSE, so when we faced especially difficult situations, there was no relationship to fall back on and no one who had a full appreciation of the seriousness of the circumstances. The HSE had become a massive organisation following its emergence from the health boards and there were huge numbers of administrative staff, with hundreds at senior levels. Sometimes I wondered if a major part of the health budget was going on the administration of the health service rather than on providing direct patient care. In practical terms as more and more layers of administration were put between the clinical coalface and the body providing up to 80 per cent of our funding, it became increasingly difficult to have conversations about risk.

Every month, I would meet officials from the HSE for performance meetings, during which we fed back the Rotunda's financial information and our clinical concerns. From the officials' point of view, so long as we were within our budget, everything was fine. We were very good at measuring activity levels and we brought that information to our performance meetings, but it was glossed over. When I raised the issues and emphasised the risk, there was never any real engagement with the person I was talking to. Instead, they focused on our budget and our headcount. The country was going through a crisis in public finances, a bailout and pressure from the Troika, and there was limited money available, so the health budget was under pressure. The HSE were under instructions to make sure that everyone stayed within budget, and part of staying within budget was keeping the staffing headcount down. They had to bring information back to their seniors within the hierarchy of the HSE, who, in turn, were being instructed by the Departments of Health and of Finance. The fact that our activity levels were rising appeared to make no difference, nor did the issue of quality of service appear to be a priority. At some point someone somewhere had decided that, in relation to budget, the Rotunda needed a particular amount of money to function every year and this amount was not going to be adjusted to respond to increased numbers of patients or levels of activity.

Headcount restrictions meant that we were not even allowed to employ more clinical staff to help us get through this difficult time. Even though we had a certain amount of autonomy within our budget as a Section 38 hospital, the restrictions on the number of full-time staff were placed on us by the HSE. I almost felt that it would require a serious crisis in order to get this onto a political agenda.

In the long run, despite the lack of meaningful engagement from the HSE, thankfully we got through that period, although I felt we were sailing very close to the wind. But it showed me very clearly why voluntary hospitals, with their attitudes and ethos, are so important to healthcare in Ireland. Many of our traditional characteristics got us through that period, from the camaraderie and mutual support of the entire staff to the Board of Governors being able to use their discretion and divert private funds to help a large number of women with benign gynaecological issues who would otherwise have had to wait. The national circumstances were very difficult and the non-alignment of ethos with the HSE was very challenging. The state authorities wanted control but did not want to take any responsibility for the significant increase in risk during that time. The balance between control and risk management is absolutely one that requires partnership. They were happy for us to have the responsibility, but were reluctant to work with us to manage it.

At the time of writing in 2021, the ability of voluntary hospitals to use their discretionary funds to sort out issues may well be under threat as the HSE and the hospital groups seek to establish control over all hospital funds. There is ongoing pressure for the voluntary hospitals to accept an integrated financial management computer system with the HSE incorporating this demand in the SLAs. If this were to happen, the voluntary hospitals would lose control over their private funds and would be unable to respond to serious clinical issues in a timely manner.

10

THE MASTERSHIP:
EXPECTING THE UNEXPECTED

● ● ● ● ● ● ● ● ●

The challenges one faces during the course of the seven-year term of the mastership are varied and diverse, and, as clinicians, we are not trained for many of the situations that arise. However, having a clinician in charge ensures that patient care and clinical outcomes are always put to the fore when faced with challenging situations and decisions.

I have been fortunate to train in some great hospitals and work with some very talented and caring consultants, and this has made me aware of how important relationships at work are. During my mastership I spent a great deal of time and energy trying to make sure everyone in the hospital was valued and included in as many social activities as possible. We have a great tradition in the Rotunda of social events, such as the summer barbecue, the Christmas panto (where the juniors are encouraged to slag off the consultants), dinner dances, balls, the regular ski trip, and an inter-hospital maternity golf match where we take on the Coombe and Holles Street. Part of being a successful leader is bringing people along on the journey with you, and for me these events were a very good way of creating and maintaining team spirit. I also encouraged the tradition of the lunch culture, which had created such a supportive collegiate atmosphere over generations by allowing colleagues to chat about issues informally.

Managing the media was another big change for a new master, and the demands on my time increased as various high-profile issues arose in maternity units around the country. It was a steep learning curve; there were some journalists who were genuinely interested in the story or the issue, but there were others who only wanted a sound bite for the next day's headline or news cast. I learned very quickly who to trust and who to avoid. As the spokesman for the Rotunda, I spent a lot of time answering questions, mostly on the radio, as this was the platform I found easiest to deal with. Despite some of these interactions with the media being a bit stressful, many were good to do and interesting, and I particularly enjoyed my early morning interviews on Newstalk breakfast. Media interviews provided opportunities to show the true value of a well-run voluntary hospital and allowed us to stress the importance of good governance and oversight close to the coalface. Even the organ retention issue demonstrated how a hospital, by being transparent about its flaws, could fundamentally improve its governance so this could not happen again.

Other issues which grabbed significant media attention included the legislation around abortion and protection of life in pregnancy. My role was to explain the issues to the public and to represent the views of the hospital. I also appeared in front of the Oireachtas Health Committee to assist them in coming up with recommendations in relation to the Protection of Life During Pregnancy Bill 2013; there

I had to ensure that I gave the facts and a view that would allow for legislation to permit us to support women in their choices, while keeping my personal opinion to myself.

***

Arising out of the organ retention story, we realised that we had to take a close look at every element of the hospital's activities, and see how well governance was working and whether it could be improved. The HARI unit was one of those we examined closely. Although it was an integral part of the hospital, it was based in a discrete building on the Rotunda grounds and had been operating as if it were a separate unit. The unit had been established and run by Robert (Robbie) Harrison (1940–2017). Robbie had great qualities, but he was not the easiest man to deal with and for years the board had probably shied away from challenging him and did not fully understand what was happening there. He had since retired and, as the board was responsible for the unit, it was time to assess the governance model in detail.

Robbie had been born in England and studied medicine at the RCSI. After working in Queen Charlotte's Hospital in London as a specialist registrar with a particular interest in fertility, he returned to Dublin, where he practised obstetrics in the Rotunda and taught in TCD. His first IVF procedure was in St James's Hospital in 1985, less than a decade after the birth of Louise Brown in Britain, the world's first test-tube baby. Robbie served on the World Health Organization task force on infertility in the 1980s and was active in international obstetric organisations. In 1989, as a professor of obstetrics and gynaecology, he set up the HARI unit at the Rotunda. As head of this unit, he oversaw the births of about 4,000 babies using the developing technologies of assisted human reproduction. He retired in 2005.[1]

I was a senior house officer and on the lowest rung of the ladder when the HARI unit started up. Robbie was on call in the labour wards, so I worked with him. Although he was known as being difficult, I got on well with him, but as juniors we all recognised that he was slightly eccentric so we did not do things that would make him cross! He was totally driven, which was why he was so successful, but there was a ripple effect. While he was very well respected by many people, he was also disliked by others because he tended to step on a lot of toes. The patients appreciated him, they got a baby; and if they did not get a good outcome, they knew someone had tried very hard to help them.

Robbie retired before I took up the mastership, and the running of the HARI unit had been handed over to another consultant. When Robbie managed the unit, the figures had balanced, but there had been no visibility and no one knew what was going on there. When we examined the books, we discovered that it was actually losing money. Robbie had worked under the standard professorial agreement and, as part of that contract, a percentage of his private practice income arising from his work in the hospital had been ploughed back into the unit. But the new consultants did not have the same academic appointment, so their private income was their own. They were perfectly entitled to keep it, but it meant that the business model of the HARI unit had changed. The board decided that it could not be supported and that the easiest way to deal with it was to sell it off. In 2014 the HARI unit was sold to Virtus, Australia's largest IVF provider, and Virtus also acquired a majority ownership stake in Sims Clinic. They bought the name and rented the unit on the hospital property, so the HARI unit was no longer under the governance of the Rotunda. In 2020 the unit moved to Swords, where it became known as Sims IVF.

In the long run, ideally, IVF would be publicly funded, but as yet that has not happened. However, the board of the Rotunda sets aside some money for a small number of public patients to apply and have their IVF funded by the hospital.

***

Meanwhile, my dealings with the HSE continued to be very frustrating and there was probably a bit of attitude on both sides. I found their lack of trust and respect for the way we did things difficult. I am sure they found me equally annoying because I kept saying the same thing over and over again, stressing the clinical risks associated with high activity levels. When I talked to retired masters, they seemed to have experienced a more respectful relationship with government officials than the one I was experiencing.

The formal relationship between the Rotunda and the state was, and still is, based on an annual SLA. It was essentially a contract between ourselves and the HSE, stating that we deliver an agreed amount of services and they provide an agreed amount of funding. However, when I was master we usually signed that contract in December for the year retrospectively. The SLA was a very long document and included all sorts of things within it that we did not necessarily like, so we always ended up signing it with caveats. The HSE managed its own hospitals in every aspect, including financial, and it was as if they were trying to make us fit that mould. We kept pointing out that we had the right to our own determination and that our executive was answerable to our Board of Governors. We told them that they could not actually take the degree of control that they seemed to be demanding. They could set headcount limits and control the amount of money we received but we were still independent of them. At the same time, the split between control and responsibility was a huge problem. We had long patient waiting lists and when the HSE official said to me, 'It is your risk, you manage it,' he was ignoring the fact that the HSE was responsible for providing most of the hospital's funding. The patients on our waiting list were our responsibility and if anything went wrong, we were the ones who would be hung out to dry, not the HSE. And still our main funding body, the HSE, was not prepared to assist or even engage with the problem. Working in partnership seems to be a difficult concept for them.

As a voluntary hospital, once we had our budget, we had a certain amount of freedom so long as we did not break their rules in terms of employment numbers or go into debt. However, very often we did not know how much our funding was going to be for a given year until the end of that year. During the year we would get money in dribs and drabs to pay salaries and so on, but we would not know what the final figure was going to be until August, September or October. It made managing the hospital extraordinarily difficult. We challenged this, but little happened and it left us in a very exposed position. An HSE hospital could have a funding deficit at the end of the year and the HSE is obligated by statute to make sure that it does not run into debt. But if a Section 38 hospital runs into debt, that debt becomes its problem and leaves it in a very vulnerable position. It also meant that the HSE had the ability to squeeze the voluntary hospitals in terms of overall budget.

Interestingly we were not the only ones frustrated with the SLAs and the delayed budget. In the IRG report into the voluntary organisations,

Catherine Day and her team identified this as a significant issue for many of the voluntary hospitals, noting that the SLAs 'have become the carrier of an ever-increasing number of obligations and conditions ...'[2] The report quotes the following submission from the Voluntary Healthcare Forum:

> There is a lack of adequate and meaningful consultation in the (SLA) process for securing agreement about the SLA requirements with individual organisations. The process does not take into account unique experiences of individual service providers, such as their national specialities. Increasingly the SLA has become 'an imposed contract' which in many cases causes significant challenges for service providers.[3]

The IRG report further adds that 'There seems to be a tendency for the HSE to treat the voluntary sector as though it was part of the statutory system without taking sufficiently into account the separate legal status and private ownership of these organisations.'[4]

On the question of the budgets, the following is one of the IRG recommendations:

> We recommend a move to multi-annual budgets, initially for a 3-year period, to enable voluntary organisations to plan better and to factor innovative reform ideas and capital investment into the services they provide. This will also provide greater certainty to the State, which relies on these organisations to provide essential services.[5]

***

There were other big issues to tackle during my mastership, and one of these was the physical infrastructure. For twenty-one years or more we had been trying to get capital funds from the government to develop the hospital structurally. Our building was old, overcrowded and inadequate. Infrastructure is part of what enables ongoing improvement and innovation within a hospital, so it must be supported and continually upgraded. If we are going to run a quality organisation, get good outcomes, attract quality staff and support them in their endeavours then we need an infrastructure that is constantly supported and continually improved.

In 2011 a section of the old lath and plaster ceiling collapsed over a busy corridor. No one was injured, but it was an indication of the conditions in which we were working. Extensive renovations were not possible as we had nowhere to decant our patients, and no alternative space to carry on with our clinics. We had the necessary land on which to build a new extension, as we still own the Parnell Square site, except for the piece occupied by the Garden of Remembrance, which we had given to the state. But we needed capital investment to contruct, ideally, a major four-storey-over-basement building on the west side of the square. Peter McKenna had started the process of lobbying government for its support, Mike Geary continued it, and I picked it up when I took over. But in a recession it was difficult, not least because the new facilities would require additional ongoing expenses to pay for the services. More significant, however, was the government's intention of co-locating us, which meant that a new building on the Parnell Square site was not considered to be a useful allocation of resources. Yet while it was important to keep the need for an extension on the table, there were so many moving targets to work with that it was not an optimistic situation. Agendas needed to coalesce, including political, economic and social, for anything to move forward. We were working in an environment where there had been a huge amount of change and under the new national health structure we had no opportunity to build the necessary relationships to make this happen.

At the time of writing, the issue of providing the Rotunda with more space on Parnell Square has made some progress. The master, Fergal Malone, has moved the discussion about a new building on the west side of the square to a more advanced stage than in the past. In addition, the HSE has agreed that the Rotunda can rent Parnell House, consisting of refurbished premises from numbers 13 to 18 on the east side of Parnell Square, so we can transfer some of the hospital's activity. This will allow us to move some outpatient and administrative functions out of the current building.

***

While the relationship with the state authorities was frustrating, within the hospital we were always conscious of giving people the opportunity to come up with new ideas. Ideas for change come from all directions: young consultants, pathologists, clinicians and others who are mad with enthusiasm to change and improve things. Brian Cleary, our chief pharmacist, recently wrote, 'The innovative ethos of our founder Bartholomew Mosse lives on in the agility and innovative approach of the Rotunda Hospital. This stimulates rather than stifles creative solutions to everyday problems. Staff are encouraged to help develop hospital strategic and operational plans and can shape and influence the future direction of the organisation.'[6]

Often their ideas are not realistic, but with access to the master, at least they have a chance of airing their views. If, in my opinion as master, I believed an idea had merit, the proposer was encouraged to produce a business plan and then we could see where we could take it. One of the most innovative ideas came from our general services manager, Ray Philpott, who wanted to make the hospital more energy efficient. The HSE was calling on ten or fifteen hospitals to change their electric systems to a more efficient, cheaper and greener way of doing things. Ray heard about it, talked to them, gathered information and then approached me. He wanted us to volunteer to be one of the first hospitals to undertake a complete renovation of our electrical and generator systems. Secretary General Manager Pauline Treanor and myself looked into it and agreed to go for it. It was a way the hospital could show leadership. It was a huge amount of work, but we got a new generator, new electrical systems, changed all of the lighting in the hospital to low voltage lights and became much more energy efficient. It was funded by Sustainable Energy Ireland and in the long run savings have been generated.

Maintaining an environment that supports innovations and new ideas helps to make hospitals competitive in the packages that we offer young doctors. For them it is not just about salary but also about a hospital's services, operating theatre lists and the ability to practise what they learned during their training years at home and abroad. Within the Rotunda we have worked hard to maintain the interest and enthusiasm of our team, so that innovations and changes would be made to the benefit of the hospital and our patients, and that has allowed us to attract terrific people to our staff.

One of the great appointments made for the Rotunda during my mastership was Dr Richard Drew as consultant microbiologist in 2014. Mary Cafferkey, the outgoing consultant microbiologist, and the team in the laboratory area helped design the job description. When Richard applied, we could see he had real energy, drive and commitment, and ideas on how things could be done and done better. His desire to innovate, make changes and improvements have flourished in the Rotunda, where foresight, understanding, advanced planning and the collegiate environment allow someone with his abilities to develop services that help our patients.

A significant new appointment was Fionnuala Ní Áinle, a consultant haematologist, who was jointly appointed with the Mater to look after our haematology patients. Her appointment meant that we could provide multidisciplinary care for those challenging patients. Brian Cleary was appointed chief pharmacist and took our pharmacy to a whole new level. The expansion of Sharon Cooley's job was another very significant development and linked in with my intention to build our clinical audit and research department. Sharon was already a consultant obstetrician and gynaecologist in the hospital when we added lead audit clinician to her role. It put clinical audit on a formal footing within the hospital. Clinical audit is a very important part of understanding the outcomes of what we do. If we are going to do something new or different, introduce a new policy or a new way of doing things, we need to monitor it to see what effect the change has made. Through auditing, we can see if we need to tweak or change something, we can see what the trends are, and see if something needs to be repeated. By having a clinical audit department, we track our audits and can repeat them if necessary. It gives junior doctors an opportunity to do clinical audit when they come to the hospital. And we can see how our hospital is performing.

The ability of our voluntary hospital to attract and employ world-class staff has paid off in spades. During the Covid-19 pandemic and the 2021 cyber-attack, these staff, all of the highest calibre, have contributed hugely to our ability to respond and deal with the massive assaults on our system. Huge credit is due to Richard Drew and John O'Loughlin in the laboratory, to Brian Cleary in the pharmacy and to their teams for the way in which these issues were successfully managed.

***

Just after I took up the mastership, I found myself in Minister for Health Mary Harney's office trying to change her mind on what we considered a bad decision concerning a plan to move the analysis of smears out of the country as part of a new national cervical screening service. We wanted to keep the cervical screening service in Ireland for several reasons – financial, jobs, training and most importantly oversight. In the early 2000s, we were gearing up to be players in providing a national cervical screening service. The Rotunda's laboratory team wanted to be involved, being a very progressive and talented group of people who had pushed the boat out and planned ahead in terms of the full range of pathology services that we provided. We were already doing opportunistic screening of our own patients and, when the idea of a national screening programme came up, we wanted to be part of it. We invested heavily in the equipment required to analyse smears in much larger numbers to ensure we would have the capacity to participate in a national service. When we put in our bid we never thought that the service would leave the country. Although it was known that the Rotunda and the Coombe were ready and able to provide the service, Minister for Health Harney essentially pulled the plug and gave the contract to a company in the United States. I led a deputation from the Rotunda to advise her that this decision could prove to be a serious mistake.

Minister Harney, Dr Grainne Flannelly, gynaecologist in Holles Street and clinical lead for the new cytology service, and Tony O'Brien, who later became the director general of the HSE, were at the meeting. The three of them sat on one side of the table, while Rotunda consultant pathologists John Gillan and Dr Eibhlis O'Donovan were with me on the other. We explained to the minister that taking the service to America was a bad decision because their oversight and their governance of screening systems were completely different and not appropriate for Ireland. I explained that their levels of quality control were different; they used different terminology to report results; a good screening system requires communication between cytology, pathology and clinicians, but working across different time zones was bound to create problems; we would have no oversight or control over the governance of the system; and we would lose jobs, lose our ability to train cytology and laboratory staff, and lose skills and training opportunities as a result of the decision. In my view it was indefensible, and I said so. I believe the service was outsourced to the United States for financial reasons, as it appeared that it was going to be cheaper to buy in bulk from an existing market than set up new services within the Irish hospital network.

The contract going abroad to the United States opened a whole chapter of issues that might never have happened if the service had been under the governance of the Rotunda or the Coombe or both, because there the masters would have had ultimate responsibility for the service and a solid governance structure would have been in place. But by outsourcing the service to the United States, we lost control of oversight and governance. A board should have been appointed to oversee and control the service, but no proper governance structure was put in place. We had no control over laboratory accreditation and no oversight over quality control. The smears were being sent into a different screening system with different governance structures and there was outsourcing within that system without our knowledge.

In 2018 the government approved the establishment of a Scoping Inquiry into the CervicalCheck Screening Programme, to be undertaken by Dr Gabriel Scally, Professor of Public Health at the University of the West of England and the University of Bristol. He found that there were all sorts of issues that were not understood or were not dealt with appropriately. And then, as we know, the government had to devote huge amounts of money and personnel to an area after it became a big political issue and a terrible personal tragedy for many women and their families.

***

Another major issue that arose during my mastership was brought to light by the death of Savita Halappanavar as a result of complications of a septic miscarriage in October 2012 in University Hospital Galway.[7] Arising out of a European Court of Human Rights ruling in 2010, there had been some movement by the government to open the sensitive debate on termination of pregnancy. Savita's case raised public awareness around the issue even further. Following her death, the HSE launched an inquiry as the government discussed legislation. The inquiry found that there had been inadequate assessment and monitoring, failure to offer all management options and a failure to adhere to established clinical guidelines.[8] It made several recommendations, including legislative and constitutional change.[9]

Meanwhile the Oireachtas was holding days of discussions with relevant professionals. Jerry Buttimer TD was chairing the Health Select

Sub-Committee to discuss the Protection of Life During Pregnancy Bill 2013 and I was asked to go in and talk about the Rotunda's experience in this area. The committee was large and there was a huge amount of interest in the subject. Sticking your head above a parapet on such emotive and sensitive issues was a dangerous thing to do, as it would have been too easy to say something off the cuff, or rub people up the wrong way. At that time the only people who were speaking out were on the extremes of the argument. People in the middle were not talking about it because they were afraid of being shot down.

On termination of pregnancy, I have always taken the view as a clinician and an obstetrician that it is not for us to take one side or the other, but to support women in their choice as to what they need and want to do. We give people information and counselling, let them make their choice, support them in that choice and do not judge them. As far as I can see, that is my role as an obstetrician. I also think the term pro-life is unfortunate – everyone is pro-life, especially those working in our specialty. So I went there with no agenda, neither on one side nor the other. I was there to provide information, to represent my hospital and to talk about numbers, concerns and my experiences of this particular issue, but I was not there to give my personal view.

Jerry Buttimer deserved a lot of credit for the way he chaired the committee. He treated me as an expert witness and talked to me beforehand and afterwards, making me feel as welcome as he could in surroundings that were foreign to me. The setting is intimidating and certainly took me out of my comfort zone. There were cameras, press reporters and many other people listening to what I was saying and reporting on it straight away. It was not a discussion. The format was for three or four questions to be asked simultaneously; the witness was then expected to answer each of those questions in turn and in detail.

This was an approach that I was not familiar with and for someone who was there to give an expert opinion, it was difficult. On occasion I got so engrossed in answering the first question that it was hard to remember what the fourth question was. There were people who asked questions who clearly had an agenda and were trying to make me say things in a particular way. Sometimes the question seemed more important than the answer; the enquirer simply wanted their question on record. Although it did not happen to me at that hearing, there was an instance at another Oireachtas health committee hearing where someone asked a question and then just left, which I thought was incredibly disrespectful. But at this committee, Jerry Buttimer was very helpful and if I had not answered a part of the question, he would jog my memory. It is a format that probably suits politicians, but it is intimidating for someone coming in to assist them in their role, which is what I was there to do.

What I told them was that, as a hospital, we had a very pragmatic approach to protecting life during pregnancy. When we were in a situation where we felt that the life of a woman was at risk or in danger, and treating the woman required that the pregnancy be terminated, then that was what we did. The decision was always made by two senior clinicians, usually one being the master, and if the master was not available, it would be the next most senior person – possibly a former master. But two very senior people would have been involved in that decision. The committee asked me how many times it had happened; I responded that it was six or seven times a year. They asked me how many times I thought this would be required in Ireland every year, I answered probably between twenty and thirty times. I arrived at this number by looking at the Rotunda birth rate compared to the national birth rate: we are looking after 8,000–9,000 births per year and we would come across this situation about six or seven times; nationally there are about 60,000 births per year, which suggests that these situations may happen about twenty-five to thirty times a year. It was a rough calculation off the top of my head but in fact that figure is spot on. While such incidences do not occur frequently, it is a massively important event when it does happen and there has to be good governance around it.

I looked back at the committee recordings on Oireachtas television and it was only then that I realised that while I had attempted to answer the questions that they were asking, other witnesses seemed more political and chose not to answer the questions, but instead told the committee what they wanted them to hear. I answered the questions to the best of my ability. That is the clinician in me. Every day when I am sitting down at a clinic with a woman in front of me, I am answering questions, explaining and clarifying, whether it is in relation to a decision that needs to be made or explaining what the situation is. So, my first inclination when I am asked a question is simply to answer it.

The Protection of Life During Pregnancy Act was signed into law by President Michael D. Higgins in July 2013. It defined the circumstances and processes in which a termination could be legally performed in Ireland. The issue of termination of pregnancy came to the fore again in 2017, by which stage my seven-year mastership was completed. I will look at the Rotunda's response to the repeal of the Eighth Amendment of the Constitution of Ireland in Chapter 12.

11

SHIFTING SANDS:
GOVERNMENT POLICY
AND THE HOSPITALS

• • • • • • • • •

As my time as master ended, I began to realise that the benefits of the Irish voluntary hospital network were simply not properly understood by the HSE, or by the general public for that matter. There was no lightbulb moment as such, just a series of events that suggested that the independence of remaining voluntary hospitals, including the Rotunda, was under threat. With the disappearance of a number of Dublin's voluntary hospitals, it seemed to me that rapidly changing governmental policy was being implemented without the implications being fully understood. There is an argument that a smaller number of large teaching hospitals with a concentration of specialised services would be more cost efficient, but at what cost? Bigger does not always mean better and it does not always mean more efficient. The governance of bigger organisations always focuses on the finances, while the smaller voluntary hospitals were locally managed with boards of management who could make cost savings, focus on the patients' needs and make rapid decisions.

During my mastership government policy changed quite quickly without the implications of the changes being fully understood. From our point of view, it was frustrating trying to work out what was going on and how we should deal with fast-moving situations. The big change came in 2013, when Minister for Health James Reilly introduced hospital groups. This had major implications for our relationship with the Mater Hospital and introduced a new layer of bureaucracy between us and the government. Going forward, our funding would come through the RCSI Hospital Group, which was set up in 2014 and formalised in 2015. In 2021 it still did not have a legal status.

Meanwhile the change of government altered the path of the New Children's Hospital (NCH), removing us from the possibility of a superb tri-located facility on the Mater site. We had been planning a possible co-location with the Mater and had nurtured our relationship with that hospital, making numerous joint appointments to help us deal with our most complex patients. But then it was decided that the NCH was going to the St James's Hospital site and the Coombe was going to be the tri-located maternity hospital, although no usable space on the St James's site has ever been allocated for that.

***

In the 1980s there were numerous voluntary hospitals in Dublin all providing services and many have gone – relocated and merged, their identities subsumed into statutory hospitals. I was an intern in Jervis Street Hospital when it was moved to Beaumont. Working in a brand-new hospital should have been a positive experience, but I found it uncomfortable and was relieved to return to the voluntary sector six months later. In 1998, the Meath, the Adelaide and the National Children's Hospital were merged to become the new hospital in Tallaght, and at that time all three hospitals were strongly represented on the new hospital board. Their initials, AMNCH, were associated with the hospital. However, this changed in 2014, when a few problems prompted the minister for health to appoint a new board with only one member from each of the original hospital boards included. The hospital was renamed the Tallaght University Hospital in 2019.[1]

The disappearance of these old voluntary hospitals is a loss, and they have been replaced by big institutions that soak up huge amounts of administrative money, but I am not sure what we have gained. Gordon Linney, Archdeacon of Dublin and an active member of our board for many years, was a member of the AMNCH board in Tallaght. He told the story of how the HSE responded to a major cost saving when the original board was in charge:

> Tallaght has a big orthopaedic facility. We were funded to do a large number of hip replacements per year. We were absolutely delighted when we did nearly 40 per cent more than expected. But the HSE reaction was to cut our budget. The orthopaedic team had improved the service and had done a brilliant job, and the reward was that their budget was cut on the basis that they were obviously getting too much money.[2]

***

In 2008, there was talk about a possible tri-location of the Rotunda with the Mater and Temple Street Children's Hospital (TSCH), and this continued during my mastership. The proposal to rebuild TSCH on the Mater campus had been around for some time – I had heard talk about it when I came back from London in 1996. Minister for Health Mary Harney had the idea that co-location of hospitals was the way forward. In 2005 the HSE engaged McKinsey and Co. to advise on the provision of paediatric care nationally. A year later their report recommended the creation of a national children's hospital co-located with an adult acute teaching hospital and the Mater site was selected. The 2008 KPMG *Independent Review of Maternity and Gynaecology Services in the Greater Dublin Area* (KPMG report) looked at moving each of the three Dublin maternity hospitals to co-locate with an acute general hospital. None of the maternity hospitals in Dublin have an adult intensive care unit, so when our patients get very sick and require intensive care, they have to be transferred to the local adult hospital. KPMG examined various different possibilities and suggested that the Rotunda be co-located with the Mater, that Holles Street be co-located with St Vincent's Hospital, and the Coombe be co-located with either St James's Hospital or Tallaght Hospital.

We were very keen for TSCH to be moved to the Mater site because, as the closest maternity hospital to the new hospital, we envisaged a tri-location and the opportunity to have the complete package of health care from pregnancy and neonatology right through to geriatrics all on one site. It had exciting potential. Alan Ashe, the chairman of our board, worked with the chairs of the Mater and Temple Street boards to push that agenda. Given the proximity to us, we had spent many years fostering links with the Mater and had a very good working relationship with them. All of our anaesthetic consultant appointments, for example, were jointly held with the Mater, and over the years we have sent critical cases requiring acute hospital care there. Our patients had to go by ambulance, which was not ideal because it usually separated a mother from her baby. We looked forward to an arrangement where we could put a patient on a trolley, wheel her down a corridor, open a door and go straight into a new setting where there would be specialist care and specialist diagnostics.

People have different understandings of what co-location actually means. We saw co-location as geographically moving the hospital to a site near another hospital but maintaining our governance structures and our independence. There would be an opportunity to share certain services and there would be a campus governance arrangement, but the clinical governance of the hospital would have remained as it was and our voluntary status would be maintained. That was our vision for co-location. It was not to be an opportunity for the Mater to take over the Rotunda; it was to be two voluntary hospitals moving on to the same site while maintaining their clinical governance structures. As the Mater Hospital was established by the Sisters of Mercy and maintained a Roman Catholic ethos, some procedures, such as sterilisations, would not have been allowed by them at the time, but we would have looked after patients requiring such procedures at the Rotunda, so it was not an issue.

Bi-location or tri-location would require the Rotunda to move out of Parnell Square, something a lot of people in the hospital would not have been comfortable about. There is a feeling of enormous positivity and love for the old hospital. It has the atmosphere of a single speciality hospital where everybody is pulling together in the same direction and it is all about good outcomes for mothers and babies. There was certainly an anxiety that by moving to a newer and more modern setting on the campus of another hospital, we might lose some of our identity and some of those positive intangible things that we have on the site here. But there was also a recognition that modern-day care of patients has to happen and that it is no longer acceptable to have ten or twelve beds in Nightingale-style Victorian wards with no privacy, no proper storage and where infection control is a problem. A new hospital should be much easier to clean and manage, and infection rates should be lower. There would also be additional medical, surgical and intensive care support services on hand, which would make the delivery of the service safer and more efficient.

But, after all the meetings, all the negotiations and all the work, the plans for the new hospital were rejected by An Bord Pleanála in 2012. The height of the proposed structure being in excess of what the planners were willing to accept was cited as a reason for rejection, but some of us involved were not convinced that this was the only reason. There were parts of the site to which this restriction did not apply, so the designs could have been rejigged. And to be honest, if a project is so important from a national strategic perspective, those sorts of issues can be dealt with. It came down to political will at the time and there was speculation that the height was used as the excuse to reject the entire project. The story went around that the Troika, the international body overseeing Ireland's financial recovery, said that the project had to be shelved. There was also talk that the Fine Gael/Labour coalition government, which had been in power since 2011, had influenced the decision. When the NCH was originally proposed for the Mater site, Bertie Ahern had been in power and this superb facility would have been in his constituency. Ahern was also an ex-employee of the Mater.

Once it was decided that the Mater was not to be the chosen site, the Rotunda was out of the picture and we were disappointed that we were not going to be involved. It also meant that given the state of our existing facilities, we would have to look for capital investment to fund a new west wing for the hospital. Ironically, we are now in a situation where the costs of developing the NCH on the St James's site are far greater than they would have been had it been tri-located with the Mater and the Rotunda.

In 2012, a working group chaired by Frank Dolphin produced a report outlining the options. In November of that year, the government chose to build the new children's hospital on the St James's campus site. The choice of the site and the design of the NCH at St James's are going to raise all sorts of issues in time. I cannot see the Coombe moving to the site in the near future because it is very cramped and they are hamstrung in terms of what they can do.

Meanwhile the Rotunda's future is still strongly linked in with the Mater and it is our job to try to maximise those links for the best clinical outcomes for our patients. We also still have strong clinical links with Temple Street. Most of our neonatologists are jointly appointed between the Rotunda and Temple Street or Crumlin, which allows for continuity for those patients. Babies born prematurely require developmental follow up, and jointly appointed people treat those patients over a longer period of time in those clinics. By the time the NCH eventually opens, it will not be big enough or fit for purpose for all that it is expected to do. Whether they keep part of Temple Street open remains to be seen. The NCH already has a children's ambulatory department in Connolly Hospital. From our point of view, some of our neonates go to Temple Street for imaging – CT or MRI scans – but that is not so much of an issue because they go by ambulance and being transported an extra kilometre or two will not make a difference. Where the big issue will arise is with our paediatricians who are cross-appointed between the two hospitals. Currently they walk up and down from one hospital to the other to do their clinics and provide services in both hospitals, so proximity is important for the closeness of the relationship. If the two are divided by a busy city, it makes it harder to work on that relationship. The additional consideration is of course separating mothers from their sick newborn babies who require transfer to specialist paediatric services, which is not an ideal situation.

***

The hospital group initiative announced in May 2013 by Minister James Reilly meant that every hospital, regardless of governance, was to be organised into one of several networks based on principal academic links. Hospital groups based on academic links would work well in Galway, Cork and Limerick, where the academic associations and the geography of the hospitals all sit together. But in Dublin it was different. Geographically the Mater should have been part of the RCSI Hospital Group, but it was put into a group with St Vincent's Hospital, Holles Street and University College Dublin (UCD) on the south side of the city. This was because the Mater's academic links are with UCD and it would have been reluctant to lose this affiliation. The Coombe was linked with TCD and St James's Hospital, while we were placed in the RCSI Group with Beaumont Hospital, Cavan General Hospital, Connolly Hospital, Louth County Hospital, Monaghan Hospital and Our Lady of Lourdes Hospital in Drogheda. Unofficially we were referred to as the North East Group, but the RCSI wanted to use its name in the title of the group. Although I am a graduate of the RCSI and have a very strong allegiance to the university, I felt that it would be better to use a geographic name because it is likely that in the longer term the Mater will almost certainly be involved with the group because of the catchment area. Yet the Mater is a very proud UCD hospital and would have great difficulty in aligning itself with the RCSI. I argued, but it was one of the battles I lost. I still think I was right to hold out for a geographic name because now, with the realignment of hospital groups into regions, the Mater should be part of it and the name will potentially hold it back.

The idea of hospital groups arose from the work of Professor John Higgins and his *Report on the Establishment of Hospital Groups as a transition to Independent Hospital Trusts*. It became government policy and remains so at the time of writing. Higgins, who is an obstetrician and gynaecologist in Cork University Maternity Hospital (CUMH) had spent time as a registrar in the Rotunda when I was in England, so I never worked with him. He went to Australia, did subspecialist training there and returned as a consultant to CUMH. As a strong character, he would have driven his agenda with determination. It seems odd that, as a former Rotunda staff member but now in an HSE hospital, he suggested that these groups were put in place without the necessary thought going into how they were actually going to function with independent voluntary hospitals involved. Was he envisaging the slow dissolution and disembowelment of the voluntary system by it being gradually subsumed into the group system? His report seemed to suggest that the voluntary boards would cede their legal responsibility or obligations to the group, and that would happen without any engagement with the voluntary hospital boards. This is an extraordinary position and offers an insight into the failure of the state to understand the governance structure and the benefits of the voluntary hospitals.

In practical terms the groups made little difference to me when I was master. By 2013 our really high activity levels had settled down a bit and we had come to realise that we were going to have to manage any issues by ourselves. Our budget now came through the hospital group, which was an evolving structure and did not have any statutory power, and the Rotunda's own governance has not been accommodated by the group. However, in many ways it might well have suited the HSE; they would have been looking for a way to manage the voluntary hospitals and did not know how to do it, and perhaps thought this was an opportunity. Nevertheless, there is a section in the Higgins report that suggests that the model that is being proposed may not be applicable to the maternity hospitals and may have to be revisited.[3]

In summer 2015, Minister for Health Leo Varadkar announced that the Rotunda was to co-locate with Connolly Hospital in Blanchardstown.[4] In 2008, the KPMG report into maternity services in Ireland had considered a co-location of the Rotunda with Connolly but had dismissed this option because it believed it to be inappropriate. Connolly Hospital, on the outer western fringes of Dublin, did not have the range of facilities or expertise that is required to look after our seriously ill patients. Yet in just a few years after the KPMG report was published, Connolly became the co-location hospital for the Rotunda, while Holles Street co-locates with St Vincent's and the Coombe co-locates with St James's. It was a political decision and Minister Varadkar seemed keen that the agenda with Connolly Hospital was pushed. It has created a strange situation, because it still does not have services or facilities at the level required to support the Rotunda, yet continues to be part of government policy. The announcement pushed us further away from the Mater. There would have been plenty of people in the Mater who were very supportive of the Rotunda. However, the reality was that when the hospital groups were announced, and UCD, St Vincent's and the Mater were brought together with Holles Street as their maternity hospital, people in the Mater started to think that maybe their links should be with Holles Street rather than with the Rotunda. Yet we still needed to get sick patients to the best quality hospital with the best diagnostics and services, and those would not be available in Connolly until it was upgraded to a level four acute hospital, which is unlikely to happen in the near future. It was frustrating and difficult, but we had to maintain our existing clinical pathways with the Mater to care for our sickest patients. In 2021 the special arrangement between the Rotunda and the Mater continues, and we work very hard to maintain our clinical links, despite each hospital being in a different group.

***

In 2021, eight years after they were created, the governance of the hospital groups is still problematic. It was planned that each hospital group would have a CEO, a board and a chair. However, the development of each group went at a different pace. The CEOs of most of the hospital groups did not have a legal footing and, until their boards were in place, they did not have anyone to report to, apart from someone in the HSE. This was probably the wrong way to do it. The RCSI Group got their first CEO in 2014, their second in 2015 and then, in 2016, Ian Carter, already CEO of Beaumont Hospital, was appointed as the RCSI Group CEO. Beaumont is the major university hospital in our group and there is automatically a conflict of interest as we all struggle to have our budgets sorted out. Peter McKenna, former master of the Rotunda and clinical director for the HSE's NWIHP observed:

> An anomaly within the HSE is that the hospital groups are headed up by people called group CEOs. They probably should be called group managers rather than CEOs because their job

is to manage the groups. Calling them CEOs gives them the opportunity to behave as if they have independent empires, which was never really envisaged. This has nothing to do with their ability or their management grade but really they should all be managing according to one script rather than be let devise their own scripts.[5]

The chair of our Board of Governors represents the Rotunda on the RCSI Group board. From an organisational point of view, if services can be organised regionally, then decisions can be made locally that benefit the patients. However, the trouble is that hospital group boards are still too far away from the coalface to be able to make sensible decisions and I fear all they will do is control a budget.

***

As the development of the RCSI Hospital Group picked up some momentum and we started to have an input into the maternity services in Drogheda and Cavan, the two hospitals in our group with maternity units, it soon became apparent that we needed a clinical director of obstetrics and gynaecology for the group and it needed to be a Rotunda person. I did not think that I, as master, should formally take on that role because it did not come with any executive power within the group and I was very clear that my responsibility was to the Rotunda first and foremost. Former master Peter McKenna was about to retire and I was happy for him to take on an advisory role in Cavan and Drogheda, and to collect information and help them with clinical risk and so on.

At the time there was no clearly defined role for a group clinical director. There were no guidelines to say what the relationship of the clinical director was within the group or with each of the different hospitals, and there was nothing about how they might relate to the HSE hospitals, as opposed to a voluntary hospital. There was also no legal basis for them, yet clinical directors carry a threat to the autonomy of the voluntary hospitals in that they could erode the hospitals' clinical independence. As the groups evolved, each one worked it out for themselves, defining the role slightly differently.

Although there was no formal relationship between clinical leads and the group, we created the Serious Incident Management Forum (SIMF) while I was master. The idea behind it was to manage clinical risk and to raise standards across the group. Clinical risk is about learning from issues as they arise in a timely manner. It is about turning a review around to make recommendations, and it is about disseminating the information that comes from that review. By creating a review committee within the group, we thought that we could assist the other maternity units. Peter McKenna, as group clinical director of obstetrics and gynaecology, chaired that group.

The SIMF worked quite well initially because everybody brought their concerns to the forum, aired clinical issues, and discussed what we had learned and what we had done about such concerns. We developed a good understanding of what was going on in each hospital and we knew, for example, what the different hospitals' caesarean section rates and perinatal mortality rates were. These figures are published within the group on a monthly basis. But what emerged fairly quickly was that the three hospitals were using the SIMF for slightly different reasons. We had good clinical risk management in the Rotunda, so we were bringing the results of our reviews to share and discuss because it was the right thing to do. Cavan and Drogheda, however, were bringing their issues and concerns to the group to find out what sort of review we thought they should do. They were looking for decisions, whereas we were sharing information.

There were many reasons why the maternity units in Cavan and Drogheda responded to the SIMF in this way. They were smaller units with a smaller number of people involved. If there are only three or four consultants, it might be harder to do an in-depth review of a colleague. As well as that, in rural areas there is a greater degree of public scrutiny by the local community and that community might not trust the people in the hospital to review their own situation. So the maternity units needed a certain amount of outside input to validate the situation and to confirm that their decision-making was in order, and the SIMF was being used for external reviews. In the Rotunda we can say that we have been externally audited and benchmarked by independent assessors, and we can stand over our decisions. Cavan could now say that they had taken issues to the group. But the SIMF was there for assistance in terms of the options open to us, what was acceptable and what in-depth review needed to happen. Fergal Malone, when he succeeded me as master of the Rotunda, took over the role of obstetrics and gynaecology clinical director for our group from Peter McKenna. He, too, held the view that SIMF was a forum to be used as a method of upping standards and for sharing learnings from serious incident reviews across the group.

***

Despite their various problems, the positive aspects of the hospital groups have been growing steadily. During my mastership we got the concept of hub-and-spoke services off the ground in both neonatal transport and regional perinatal pathology. Foetal medicine services soon followed the same pattern, allowing both Our Lady of Lourdes Hospital in Drogheda and Cavan General Hospital to benefit from these specialist services. In recent years the amount of time the Rotunda has spent linking up with Cavan and Drogheda has increased significantly, and we work together very effectively within the hospital group, looking after the maternity, newborn and gynaecology patients in the group catchment area. We share information and expertise, and arrange training and rotations between the hospitals. Consultants are jointly appointed to enable specialist maternity services to be provided to Drogheda and Cavan in situations where they cannot appoint a full-time person to deliver those services. For example, Cavan advertised a foetal medicine position to oversee an anomaly screening service, but no one applied. So we appointed a consultant, giving that person all of the advantages of working in the Rotunda but asking them to go to Cavan and spend one day a week there overseeing anomaly screening.

In 2016 we established an Outpatient Hysteroscopy Clinic in Connolly to see gynaecology patients more quickly and to reduce waiting lists. The consultants provided examination, assessment and treatment in one facility and in one visit, removing the need for patients to make multiple visits to the hospital. To do this we took over an unused ward in Connolly and put in equipment and staff to run the clinic several days a week. It was a Rotunda clinic in Connolly under the governance of the Rotunda. When Covid hit, Connolly needed the space, so we brought the service back to the Rotunda.

Recently there has been a new initiative between the Rotunda, Drogheda and Cavan in respect of perinatal pathology services. The regional maternity units do not have sufficient numbers to justify a full-time perinatal pathologist's appointment. So Noel McEntagart was appointed to the Rotunda, but with responsibility for the services in Cavan and Drogheda too. He now works alongside our perinatal pathologists, as well as providing regional services. This arrangement enables him to keep up to date on current practice while providing the services that are required in Cavan and Drogheda. We have also established a regional neonatal transport service and a regional perinatal pathology service. Newborn babies, very premature babies and babies with problems born in Cavan, Drogheda and nationwide are transported to the Rotunda for specialist care. Ideally the mother is moved to the most appropriate hospital before the birth, but sometimes she gets delivered elsewhere and needs to be transported to the city. The neonatal transport system has a dedicated neonatal ambulance and dedicated neonatal staff. Sometimes the mother comes with the newborn, but it depends on her situation as she could be post-operative. That regional transport system has worked well.

Overall, while we have taken on a role in assisting with monitoring clinical risk and with the investigation of clinical incidents, we do not have any executive power or responsibility when it comes to managing those services in the other group hospitals, except in the case of the Connolly gynaecology clinic, where those involved are all our own staff. The maternity units in Cavan and Drogheda are part of a general hospital and those hospitals have their own administration, which ultimately leads back to the group and then back into the HSE. The governance in a situation like this should have been thought about before the groups were created. With some of the groups containing both voluntary and HSE hospitals, the governance arrangements over these hub-and-spoke services are unclear. The consultants working in these services are employees of a voluntary hospital providing a service in an HSE hospital over which the voluntary hospital, its master and its board have no jurisdiction.

The relationships between the voluntary hospitals and HSE hospitals within a group have the potential to deliver really good services to regional populations, but as we move forward into the next phase in the evolution of our health system, these relationships need to be well thought out and then put on a better footing, recognising the role and the importance of the voluntary hospital in the national system. This would improve care and outcomes, and possibly even save money by focusing on the importance of culture within the health service. At the moment the culture is about managing resources and not necessarily about improving care or providing an atmosphere and environment of innovation. However, if the role and importance of the voluntary hospital model is recognised, we may well be able to improve outcomes and develop a culture of quality improvement, innovation and everything that is good within a high-quality health care system.

***

In 2021, at the time of writing, the whole idea that the Rotunda would co-locate with a general acute hospital is still government policy, but it is a long, long way from being a reality. Connolly Hospital would have to be remodelled and significantly upgraded, the cost of which would be enormous. It would mean, in effect, building two new hospitals on the campus. There would have to be a governance structure in place to deal with those shared campus services and a governance structure to maintain the running of the individual institutions. Having seen what happened to the Adelaide, Meath and National Children's Hospital in Tallaght, this is going to be difficult.

One of the prerequisites of co-location is that it brings with it economies, so there would be significant pressure to share facilities and services. For example, with regard to access to theatres, any question of reducing clinical services currently under the umbrella of the Rotunda would be very much a deal-breaker when it comes to co-location. We are an obstetrics and gynaecology hospital with consultants and trainees, and we need access to the full range of our speciality services in order to maintain our status as a teaching hospital. We cannot have a situation where our gynaecology services are just absorbed into the general hospital, especially as they are one of the first areas to be squeezed when a hospital is under pressure.

Sharing some services, such as maintenance, security and waste, would be straightforward. But sharing others, such as catering, might not be good for the Rotunda. The Rotunda Hospital catering service is legendary for the quality of its food. We provide probably the best patient food in the city and the role our catering team plays in maintaining the camaraderie and sense of community among staff is not to be underestimated. For staff, consuming food is an integral part of the day, a chance to unwind, to talk about the difficult delivery, to share experiences and to relax. In any hospital co-location, catering is one of the first services to be merged and if that were to happen to the Rotunda, I would see this as a big concern and a huge loss. When the Richmond and Jervis Street were moved to Beaumont, the quality of food fell off the cliff face and no one used the restaurant. If our catering facilities were to be merged on a big campus, we would no longer have the intimate and supportive ambience that our current Rotunda catering facilities afford us.

Then there is the question of service development. What the voluntary hospitals have is a culture of strategic thinking, strategic development and service planning that is done effectively at a local level and delivered in a collegiate manner. HSE hospitals in the main do not have that culture, that expectation or that experience. As a voluntary hospital, our expectation is that we are going to be strategic, innovative and adapt to the needs of our patients. I have no doubt but that the staff working in HSE institutions would embrace this culture if given the chance to do so.

***

In July 2019, Minister for Health Simon Harris announced six new geographic regions for delivering health and social care services in Ireland. Under the regional plan, the Rotunda is part of Area A, which covers Dublin north, Meath, Louth, Cavan and Monaghan, and now includes the Mater as well as Beaumont.[6] The minister indicated that the new regional authorities would have their own budgets and produce their own workforce plans to deal with specific needs in their areas, but staff pay rates would continue to be determined at central level. In launching it, Harris stated that the HSE was not fit for purpose and that the new regional approach would remove layers of managers in the health service, although no redundancy plans to reduce staffing levels within the HSE were announced.[7] And once again there was no clear plan as to how the voluntary hospitals would fit into the new arrangement.

By 2021 the only hospital group that had actually been given a legal basis was the paediatric hospital group established by the Children's Health Act 2018. In this act, two voluntary hospitals – Temple Street Children's University Hospital and Crumlin Hospital – were joined with parts of Tallaght Hospital and transferred to Children's Health Ireland (CHI). It is nominally a voluntary group, but only time will tell if the hospital holds onto the essence of its voluntary origins. In

2021, while I was writing this book, Temple Street lost its board and its CEO. Meanwhile a board and a CEO were appointed to the CHI with oversight over Temple Street. So now there is no CEO at Temple Street Hospital and therefore there is no one person on site in charge of the hospital. Governance is provided from afar by a CEO and a board whose main concern is the New Children's Hospital. This is the latest example of a situation which I believe should be avoided.

Meanwhile in terms of the future of the three Dublin maternity hospitals, the only one that has made any progress along the co-location journey is Holles Street. This has been fraught with difficulties, especially around religious aspects concerning what services can or should be provided in a co-located hospital, as well as issues around governance and ownership. Obstetrician and former master of Holles Street Peter Boylan has been very vocal in relation to this.[8] It should be a given that all women's health services which are legal within the state should be provided on this site and I think all sides have come a long way to get to a point where most people are reassured that religious beliefs will not be an issue. But there are still differing views as to whether such issues will re-emerge once the co-location has been completed.

The new hospital is going to be paid for by the state and, at the time of writing, St Vincent's Hospital Group insists that it must retain ownership of the land. There are calls for state ownership and state control of the hospital, which would put Holles Street at risk of losing its voluntary status and becoming an HSE hospital by default. This might, on the surface, seem like a good idea, but in wresting control away from St Vincent's, much of the good that comes with voluntary status will be lost. This is something that many people contributing to the public debate perhaps do not understand. What we should be striving to achieve from co-locating Holles Street with St Vincent's is an independent voluntary hospital in a co-located setting, having all the benefits of clinical autonomy, with the ability to adapt and respond to the needs of women, to attract and retain quality medical and midwifery staff, providing the best quality outcomes from a modern, world-class facility at the same time as having accountability to its independent voluntary board and the state authorities.

12

THE LATEST DEVELOPMENTS

• • • • • • • • •

I stepped down as master in December 2015 and over the following years there were several significant developments in relation to obstetrics, voluntary hospitals and the Irish health services. In 2016 the government's National Maternity Strategy was launched. In 2017 the government announced Sláintecare, which, if fully implemented, would have a negative impact on the future viability of the Rotunda and other voluntary hospitals. In 2018, the Eighth Amendment of the Constitution was repealed following a national referendum, and termination of pregnancy was then permitted by law in Ireland. And in 2019 the IRG, established by Minister for Health Harris in 2017 and chaired by Catherine Day, published its report, which shone a harsh light on the relationship between the voluntary hospitals and the state authorities, most notably the HSE.

During my mastership the government established the National Clinical Programme in Obstetrics and Gynaecology as a joint initiative between the HSE Clinical Strategy and Programmes Division and the Institute of Obstetricians and Gynaecologists in the Royal College of

Physicians of Ireland (RCPI). Michael (Mike) Turner, a former master of the Coombe, was appointed as the first National Lead on the programme in 2010 and held the position until 2019. Mike's objective was to raise standards across the country and there were lots of different ways he could have approached this. He could have conducted a clinical audit; or surveyed caesarean section rates and perinatal outcomes across different regions; or looked at the number of midwives in the unit, ratio of midwives to deliveries, or consultants to deliveries to see where there were weaknesses in the system; or the number of locums versus full-time consultants. These would have been practical, transparent, tangible changes that would have improved standards. The approach he took was to create a suite of guidelines, the National Clinical Guidelines in Obstetrics and Gynaecology. Now, following extensive consultation, the National Clinical Programme in Obstetrics and Gynaecology publishes and reviews national clinical guidelines on an ongoing basis.

Initially I was quite sceptical about this approach. Creating national guidelines and stating how we should do things sounds laudable, but problems arise if a hospital or unit does not have the facilities or the staff or the infrastructure to do something in a particular way. Then all we are doing is creating a stick to beat someone with, because the idea that anyone within the HSE was really going to listen and provide funding to ensure that the guidelines could be followed throughout the country was, in my opinion, naive.

Mike Turner was also sceptical, but in his case it was about how much he might be able to achieve in his new role. In a discussion with me, he described his experience:

[An official in the HSE] wanted me to take NHS [Britain's National Health Service] guidelines and change the headings.

I explained that this was not possible because we don't have the same resources. So I set the guidelines up from scratch, modelling them on SIGN [Scottish Intercollegiate Guidelines Network] and we had a qualifying statement, which I picked up in Queensland in Australia that said that you had to work within the resources that were available to you. That got us off the hook you are concerned about. But it was typical in that they gave us no money to do it.

We managed to get midwives and the other professionals to buy into it. My colleagues stepped up to the plate in that many of them wrote good guidelines on a pro bono basis. To give you an example, when it came to the miscarriage report, I worked closely with Bill [Professor William Ledger, now of the University of New South Wales] who was writing it. Bill and myself talked most weekends.

The guidelines have been remarkably successful. Hospitals outside the six teaching hospitals didn't have the resources to develop their own guidelines so they could trust these and apply them. In some cases practices have changed. The best example would be the miscarriage misdiagnosis, where the guidelines have eliminated problems altogether.[1]

On a number of occasions in different units, there was an issue with misdiagnosis with early pregnancy because of lack of training and a lack of good ultrasound equipment. A woman with an ongoing pregnancy may have been misdiagnosed as having had a miscarriage, perhaps in an emergency department, and may have had some sort of intervention to deal with a miscarriage, but when she was rescanned in an early pregnancy unit with a more experienced person using better equipment, it may have been found that the pregnancy was in fact ongoing. Mike continued:

We got €3 million to implement the guidelines. Working with a terrific midwife in the HSE, we did a deal with GE Healthcare on the Voluson ultrasound system. It was the machine that the obstetricians around the country wanted. The machines cost €100,000 each, but on the basis that we were going to buy one for each of the nineteen maternity units, we did a deal and got them for €65,000 each. Rather than give the saved money back to the HSE, I suggested that we use the entire budget for 27 machines, so we could give the six bigger units an extra machine. The company were very happy with the deal and we delivered value for money. But when it came to the software, the terrific midwife had moved on and the HSE insisted on controlling the negotiation. They did not get a bargain.

The national suite of clinical practice guidelines is still being developed and revised periodically by the Institution of Obstetricians and Gynaecologists with the HSE. After my initial hesitation, I agree that it is very useful to have them there and it is important that they are kept up to date.

***

The next major step in streamlining the Irish maternity services came in January 2016 when the National Maternity Strategy 2016–2026 was launched under the authority of Minister for Health Leo Varadkar. The strategy was to map out the future for maternity and neonatal care in Ireland. The chair of the National Maternity Strategy Steering Group was Sylda Langford and there were another thirty people in the steering group, so it was difficult to get consensus. There was fairly wide consultation, but the agenda was dominated by a vocal minority who wanted to keep women out of hospitals and who spoke a lot about over-medicalisation of obstetrics. The process that contributed to the National Maternity Strategy raised the issue of 'territorialism', the idea of one group of professionals having ownership over maternity services. In my opinion we need to get away from that idea: obstetrics and midwifery are complementary, and terms such as obstetric-led or midwifery-led should be parked in history. It should be about patient care by the appropriate professional. The strategy group had few obstetricians on it, yet it is important to give them an effective voice in the development of the Irish maternity health services. Although we do not claim to have all of the answers, we work at the coalface and know what is going on and what is needed. My view on it is that the midwives who manage home births were coming at it with very strong opinions, but they do not necessarily have the data, the reporting structures or the clinical governance systems to back up what they are asking for. The minority were happy with the strategy, but because of the imbalance it is not going anywhere quickly.

During the course of the discussions, there were a lot of questions about the number of maternity units around the country. Do we need nineteen maternity units in Ireland? For example, in a very small geographical area there are units in Wexford, Waterford, Clonmel and Kilkenny, and many of those would be delivering low numbers. But when you bring politics and county pride into it, are you going to allow a situation where you potentially have no babies born in Kilkenny, for example, anymore?

The implementation of the National Maternity Strategy led to the establishment of the NWIHP in January 2017. The programme was designed to lead the management, organisation and delivery of maternity, gynaecology and neonatal services across primary, community and acute care settings. Peter McKenna, former master of the Rotunda, was appointed national clinical director of the programme. Peter recalled the background to the NWIHP:

> Because the National Maternity Strategy decided that the HSE did not have sufficient oversight over maternity, the Department of Health created the NWIHP. It is an unusual situation in that the Department contacts us directly rather than goes through channels in the HSE. Initially this did not work well because we are a little bit like the cuckoo in the nest, we are employed by the HSE but we were someone else's egg, and the HSE didn't exactly know what to do with us.[2]

Nearly five years later, the health programme has struggled to fulfil its objective. Peter and his colleagues have spent most of their time dealing not with maternity but with issues arising in gynaecology, the most serious of which were CervicalCheck, mesh surgery for urinary incontinence and the outcomes of legislation legalising the termination of pregnancy, none of which were in the National Maternity Strategy. And then the Covid pandemic interfered with further developments.

There are a lot of recommendations in the National Maternity Strategy, but there have been few actions. Over the years there has been little or no interest in improving maternity and gynaecology services. It has been up to the three Dublin maternity hospitals with Cork University Maternity Hospital to drive and improve the care of women and their babies. This has been done by attracting quality staff and, despite the underfunding of the service and the failure of the HSE to recognise the poor facilities in which we work, it is because the voluntary hospitals have taken their role so seriously and delivered so well that concerns with regard to facilities have not hit the public radar. The fact that there have not been more bad outcomes is testament to the quality of the service provided by motivated and highly qualified professionals within the voluntary sector – and being voluntary hospitals, we have the freedom to attract these staff.

Mike Turner agrees:

[Maternity services in Ireland] have the lowest number of consultants in the OECD, yet our maternal mortality and perinatal mortality are very good.[3] When you look at the maternity statistics in an international context comparing us favourably with the USA and UK, which are much wealthier countries, our maternity stats hold up very well. So we are doing something right and I think the thing we were doing right is that we had very centralised services, very committed obstetricians and we have a fantastic midwifery support.[4]

In recent times, there has been a shift in the delivery of gynaecology services as they become more subspecialised. We are moving to a situation where obstetrics and gynaecology are separating and there are more people doing one or the other. Within gynaecology we are getting specialists in oncology, urology, lapocopracy surgery, endometriosis and other subspecialisations. Therefore, the demand for space, for theatre and for facilities is expanding and evolving.

Mike Turner made an interesting observation:

Kieran O'Driscoll [former master of Holles Street and advocate of Active Management of Labour] is one of my heroes in obstetrics but one of the criticisms I have of him is that he had this attitude towards obstetrics that was frugal. Everything was about low tech, keeping costs down and I think that has hurt us big time in the past because when the cuts came, they cut maternity in much the same way as they cut everything else. So to this day they have put no new funding into maternity. [Ministers for Health] Leo Varadker and Simon Harris and Stephen Donnelly talk the talk when it comes to funding maternity services. But the extra €10 million that was meant to go into the NWIPH office in 2020 was redirected into the termination service. If you want to fund the termination services, fine, but you shouldn't be redirecting money that was intended for ongoing pregnancies.

There has been some progress in recent times. Peter McKenna said, 'During 2020 we began to get a little more traction within the HSE in that they recognised that maternity and gynaecology have been dealt with badly within the HSE. All of a sudden we are getting funding through the Department of Health to set up the ambulatory gynae units, infertility hubs and so on.'

In 2021, the Rotunda benefited from Peter's work when we opened a new ambulatory gynaecology facility in the building that had been vacated by the HARI unit the previous year. The outpatient facility gave us much more space and privacy, and assisted in greatly reducing our gynaecology waiting lists. Funding to set that up came from the Rotunda and from money allocated by NWIHP to reduce waiting lists as part of the National Maternity Strategy. With the help of Peter's group and through strong clinical leadership and good project management, we were able to revamp the building and set this clinic up within three months.

***

In 2017, a cross-party parliamentary committee looking into system reform and universal health care in Ireland published a report called Sláintecare. It is a high-level policy roadmap to be phased in over a ten-year period. There are positive aspects to it, in that there is an investment in community and the possibility for many people to be treated outside the hospital setting. For many years the Rotunda has put community antenatal clinics in place to allow women to access antenatal care without having to come into the hospital. The clinics are usually based in HSE community health clinics, but the community midwives are employed by the hospital. It brings the care closer to the women's homes and makes life a little bit easier for them.

But one of the difficulties with Sláintecare is that it is proposed under this policy to take all private care out of public hospitals, including voluntary hospitals, and it is hard to see how this would function from a maternity point of view. There are no private maternity hospitals in Ireland at the time of writing. In the past there was Mount Carmel Hospital in Dublin, but it has been closed for some time. There is also no plan to introduce private maternity into the country and there probably will not be because of the clinical indemnity issue and neonatal intensive care. Yet some women will still want a choice of obstetrician, or the choice of a private room, but under Sláintecare those choices will be removed. This is going to create an income shortfall that will have to be picked up by the HSE and the government. Of the 20 to 30 per cent of income that we raise, the bulk of it comes from private patients' accommodation fees. The same would apply in other voluntary hospitals. So, if private care is taken out of these hospitals, there will be a sizeable income gap in hospital budgets. As well as that, the 20 to 25 per cent of patients who are currently paying for private facilities in the maternity hospitals will become public patients, and the work has to be done anyway, but there will be no money coming in from it.

Not being able to accommodate private or semi-private patients would reduce the ability of hospitals to attract good staff. After training abroad, part of the attraction of coming back to Ireland is that you are coming back to work in, for example, the Rotunda, where you have not only a good, well-run hospital, but you may have an element of private practice to your work as well. In addition, the consultants' vested interest contributes to high standards in everything from equipment and facilities, to food and general management, because that is what they want for their private patients in the voluntary hospital setting. If consultants are not offered the chance of engaging in some level of private practice, the package becomes less attractive, so fewer people will return. This also applies to consultants working in HSE hospitals, who may have a private practice. How the consultants manage their public and private commitments is down to them and their own ethical standards. There is an onus on the hospital to keep records of, and generate reports on consultants' activity, so if there are anomalies in a consultant's activity levels, which suggest that he or she is treating private patients at the expense of public patients, it should be picked up. In the Rotunda, this would be identified very quickly and stamped out. Colleagues, other consultants and midwives would not put up with it.

Then there is the question of renegotiating the contracts of hundreds of consultants who currently have contracts that allow them to work privately and publicly. Do you buy them out? If so, there will be significant costs and no doubt also an impact on recruitment and retention within the existing consultant body. Consultants' contracts are always a thorny issue and there is the outstanding matter of new entrant consultants being brought in on lower salaries. This inequity still has to be resolved. There is a risk that Sláintecare will turn into an argument about consultant contracts and will distract from the main purpose.

Given that Sláintecare is a complex, multi-layered programme, the term itself means different things to different people, but the focus of this wide-ranging reform should be firmly on improving the quality of patient care. The environment in which the medical and support staff work is the important bit, and not what it is called. We should be striving for better community care and better care in hospitals, and looking for ways to go about achieving that. The voluntary hospital experience clearly demonstrates that this can be done through establishing an infrastructure and creating an environment that is supportive, innovative and adaptable, in which people are happy to work. In these circumstances, people will be provided with the supports they need in their own quest to constantly improve the quality of service. So, while I think that the community side of Sláintecare is a good element and one that we were moving to anyway, I believe the overall cost of Sláintecare will prove to be too expensive. We also need to be very careful as we move to the Sláintecare model that we do not lose any of the value of the voluntary hospitals, and this is another reason why I am bringing the value and role of the voluntary hospitals to public attention.

***

Legislation concerning the termination of pregnancy in Ireland arose again in 2018. Under the Offences against the Person Act 1861, abortion was illegal in Ireland. In 1967 the British Abortion Act became law, legalising abortion there in certain circumstances. Following this, the medical social workers in the Rotunda received requests for termination from time to time, but Irish law did not permit it. Each year, thousands of women who had examined all options made their own arrangements to have legal abortions outside Ireland. The Rotunda made it clear that on their return we were there for them if they needed us. In 1983, after a bitter campaign, the country voted for the Eighth Amendment to the Constitution, which inserted a subsection recognising the equal right to life of the pregnant woman and the unborn child. Problems with this arose over the years and following continuous campaigning, a referendum was held in 2018 to repeal this amendment.

I followed the repeal campaign closely. I was always very careful to say, when anyone asked, that my personal view was not important. My job as an obstetrician is to support women in their choice. I always believed that having a termination service was very much part of a total women's health service and therefore it was an important thing to have in the hospital. However, my experience of termination was mostly in King's College Hospital in London, where there were as many terminations as there were births, and I had found that difficult. It coloured my view and I did not want to get into a situation where we would be replicating that model here.

In the Rotunda we did not know what the demand for the service was going to be, but we were pretty sure that a lot of the burden was going to have to be borne by the voluntary maternity hospitals. Our big concern was that it would become a problem on top of an already stretched service and again gynaecology lists would be squeezed. Even adding one or two surgical procedures each day would mean that one or two gynaecology procedures would have to wait. Consequently, there was a danger that we would find it difficult to provide services for our existing patients.

It also raised issues for the staff. Here we have a set of individuals who are providing a service, but they have their own beliefs, understandings and opinions. We are no different to any population of adults in that there is a spectrum of attitudes. When it came to trying to decide how we were going to manage this service, we needed people to support the women and the choices that they had made, so we asked our staff if they were prepared to be involved and under what circumstances. This included staff in outpatients and in theatre as well as senior clinicians. If someone had objections, there was no need for them to be involved, but as it happened, enough people were prepared to buy in. There were no difficulties and no one tried to impose their view on anyone else in either direction.

Another concern we had was that people might come to Dublin from around Ireland in significant numbers to avail of the service. While this service might be available in hospitals like Waterford or Cavan or Portlaoise, many of the patients would be neighbours of the people working in those hospitals and the question was whether someone would be willing to have a termination in the hospital where they might be looked after by someone they knew.

The board also recognised that it had a responsibility to maintain the welfare of staff and to reassure themselves that everything was going to be done properly. They would have sought reassurance from the master, Fergal Malone, firstly, that the hospital had the capability to deal with it; secondly, that the staff were willing to do what was being asked of them; thirdly, that there were appropriate facilities and services in place to allow the service to start up and be maintained; and finally that other people were not discommoded as a result of it.

Despites some reservations, the Rotunda agreed to go ahead with the service because we thought that it was the right thing to do and we would be ready to provide the service when the law was enacted. As it played out, much of the work was taken on by GPs who were willing to be involved in the service – and huge respect and gratitude to them, because they do it very well. A lot of the women who have terminations for non-medical reasons, have them very early, at about five to seven weeks, and this is managed without any resort to surgical termination. The number of cases that come to our door is very small. My concerns were allayed, and the service has not impacted hugely on our existing services. Our hospital has not been overrun, and I have not heard of it being an issue in other hospitals either. It has taken up some theatre and staff time, but nothing to the extent that we were worried about.

***

Amid all of the struggles with government policy and the erosion of our independence, there was a beacon of hope in 2019 with the publication of the *Report of the Independent Review Group established to examine the Role of Voluntary Organisations in Publicly Funded Health and Personal Social Services* (IRG report), which I have referred to throughout this book. The terms of reference directed the IRG to look at issues such as those arising from the provision of services through religious or faith-based organisations, the protection of public capital investment and risk management, and issues arising in the future having regard to changing patterns of religious affiliation in the population.

The review group was chaired by Catherine Day and, after a thorough process, she and her team strongly supported voluntary hospitals and voluntary organisations generally, and described how important they are in the current delivery of health services in Ireland. Their report helped to challenge a simplistic view of the voluntary sector, pointing out the legalities and the costs involved in attempting to abolish the sector and replace it with government services. The report acknowledged 'a strained relationship between the voluntary sector and the State, represented by the HSE as the funding agency'.[5] The recommendations included a rebuilding of the relationship between the state and the voluntary sector based on trust, partnership and mutual recognition of need. Overall, it seemed to be suggesting that in order to develop a system of governance for the Irish health service, the government and its agency, the HSE, needed to trust people to get on with it and allow them to deliver the kind of high-quality care that we routinely deliver in the voluntary sector.

One of the twenty-four recommendations of the IRG report was the establishment of the Dialogue Forum, to be composed of senior representatives from the HSE and its board, the Department of Health and HIQA, as well as eight voluntary umbrella organisations. Its terms of reference were about improving the relationship: 'The Forum will provide a regular platform for dialogue between the State and voluntary providers of health and social care services and will have an overarching mandate to build a stronger relationship between the State and voluntary providers for the benefit of patients and service users.'[6]

We are represented at this forum by the Voluntary Healthcare Forum (VHF), which was created by the chairs of many of Ireland's voluntary hospital boards in 2014. The VHF arose in part from a conversation

I had with our chairman, Alan Ashe, on a way to a meeting with the CEO and the board of the Mater Hospital during my mastership. With all of the pressure coming on the voluntary hospitals, we agreed that it be a good idea for the voluntary hospitals to come together and work to promote our respective interests. Out of that came the North Dublin Hospitals Group and from there came the VHF. The VHF is a high-powered group of strategists who undertake research and publications, and in a spirit of partnership engage robustly with the state to advance the delivery of excellent healthcare. There are seventeen voluntary hospitals in the VHF, including the Rotunda, the Mater, St James's and Children's Health Ireland, which has responsibility for Dublin's three children's hospitals and will run the NCH when it is completed. The VHF has commissioned research and published reports, making submissions to the state and to the IRG.

In June 2021, a document, *Building a New Relationship between Voluntary Organisations and the State in the Health and Social Care Sectors*, was published by the National Economic and Social Council based on the work of the Dialogue Forum. It drew on the experience of the healthcare sector's response to the Covid-19 crisis, citing it as an example of 'dynamic and collaborative framework in action, in real time'.[7] It noted that 'The crisis has transformed the environment in which the State and voluntary actors operate. It has also supported the transition to a new and more productive relationship, underpinned by a commitment to collective problem-solving, innovation and practical action. Equally, it has reaffirmed that mutual interdependence is a defining characteristic of Ireland's hybrid healthcare system.'[8]

The Dialogue Forum sought to build on this positive relationship by understanding how it evolved and how it can be developed for the benefit of patients and their families. In the HSE response, there was a sense that the people in the upper echelons of the health service were grateful for the coordinated response from all the hospitals and that they recognised the value of the voluntary hospital leadership during the crisis. But their response also talks about control, especially of finances and the financial model. So, although we still have a way to go, the underlying sense of the relationship is that it is warmer than in the past and hopefully this can grow.

∗∗

The Rotunda's own experience of the Covid-19 crisis, which started in March 2020, was one of disruption to the normal running of the hospital. We had to prepare for a large number of potentially infected patients and we had to protect our staff. We needed to work out how we were going to create space to segregate patients and to ascertain whether they were positive, negative or unknown. The only way we could do that was to take space from those services that could be suspended. Once again, the gynaecology lists were affected. We created a new labour ward in the antenatal ward and moved the antenatal ward to the gynaecology ward, which was evacuated. It was a matter of reshaping the service, creating new pathways and working out what we were going to do in particular clinical scenarios.

We tested people if they had symptoms; we also set up a drive-through testing system for those who contacted the hospital to say they had symptoms. We were not a Covid receiving hospital, so we had no facilities to treat people who were sick with the virus. Only those with obstetric reasons were encouraged to come to the hospital, and in that way we managed. At an early stage during the pandemic, we would have had quite a number of staff off duty because they had been in contact

217

with someone who was positive, but compared to other hospitals, our numbers were low. Within four weeks, thanks to our forward-thinking consultant microbiologist Richard Drew, we had in-house testing for the virus readily available. We were among the first hospitals to have that up and running, because we already had the equipment to run it. Here was another example of a voluntary hospital's ability to respond to an unexpected situation.

13

STEPPING DOWN FROM THE MASTERSHIP AND SOME PERSONAL REFLECTIONS

• • • • • • • • •

After my seven-year mastership was completed and Fergal Malone took over the role, I remained on in the hospital, returning to full-time obstetrics and gynaecology. Stepping down from the CEO role can create a tricky dynamic, but former masters are an enormous resource for the hospital, as the knowledge and experience gained is valuable and should not be lost. My job as master was over, but were there ways in which lessons learned could be shared within the Rotunda without interfering with the vision and work of the new master? And were there perhaps ways in which the experience gained by the outgoing master could be used constructively outside the hospital in the wider healthcare environment?

Fergal agreed that I should work on the management of clinical risk in the hospital. Major clinical incidents used to be brought to me as master, but I was aware that there was a need to disseminate information and knowledge arising from these incidents across the hospital. We had our long-standing clinical risk meetings where we reviewed issues on a weekly basis. There was also the monthly RCSI Group meeting of the SIMF. And we, of course reported our figures to the HSE at our regular performance meetings. My new role was to gather data in terms of understanding clinical risk across the hospital in obstetrics and gynaecology, and to make recommendations to Fergal about the type of review that would be required in each instance. What we were looking for were care issues that had fallen through the gaps, and systems that had not worked particularly well in a situation. We undertook to review every incident very shortly after it happened and, most importantly, to ascertain what we could learn from an adverse event and get the information back to the relevant areas of the hospital quickly so appropriate changes could be made.

Anything from one to four incidents could be brought to our regular clinical risk meetings, and when they reach this level, each one is a significant clinical incident. Minor incidents are dealt with differently. Usually, we do not need to do anything other than to record the fact that, for example, somebody charted the right medication on the wrong chart and to make sure the person was aware of the error. But a patient who has nearly died with a ruptured ectopic pregnancy is a major issue and we need to examine everything related to that incident to make sure that it does not happen again. The same group came to the meetings and included two to three consultant obstetricians, several former midwives from the clinical risk department, a consultant anaesthetist, a consultant paediatrician and a senior non-consultant hospital doctor (NCHD). It was like holding a review. Each case was presented in terms of the clinical details. The clinical risk manager recorded the outcome of our meeting, what decisions had been made, and what recommendations were made to the executive management team concerning the review that was required. Sometimes bad things happen because they just happen. They are not necessarily anyone's or anything's fault, they just happen. If everyone has done all the right things, we can look back and say that everything possible was done correctly and this is an unfortunate set of circumstances. But we need to look at everything first to be able to say that. The patient's family are given the results, although in most cases an open disclosure conversation would already have happened. In some cases, if it had not happened, we would recommend that this takes place and, if a review took place, that it was shared with the woman and her family.

As obstetricians, we are constantly aware that we are not far away from ending up in court. Our clinical meetings are fully transparent and the outcomes are accessible through Freedom of Information requests. If someone has a bad outcome and suffers some sort of harm from it, or their baby is damaged in some way, we are not unhappy for them to be compensated. For the vast majority of injuries that happen to mothers and babies, it is not anyone's fault. It is not personal, so we do not take it personally.

The Rotunda's timely review and dissemination of information process is an evolving activity within the hospital. We now have a mechanism whereby a multidisciplinary group of people – consultants, junior hospital doctors and midwives – attend weekly clinical review meetings. Each individual at that meeting is tasked with bringing back the learning or concerns that were raised to their own management forum. It is all about speed of reaction to issues as they arise – quick review, quick learning and quick change. And because we are monitoring clinical incidents on a weekly basis, we can see trends, so it enables us to advise when changes of guidelines or changes of policy are required. We cannot stop a patient having an unforeseen complication, but we can deal with it better when it does happen. We deal with healthy, well women most of the time, but sometimes a healthy woman will become sick, and recognising that is really important. So, for example, when we have a situation where we feel that the recognition was slow, we will highlight the set of circumstances around it and have an education session, led by a multidisciplinary group of junior doctors to review it, present it and learn from it. We would devote one of our regular teaching sessions to this. The midwife staff would be encouraged to attend as well as the consultants and junior medical staff. That has been a challenge during Covid because we have had to do it over Zoom. People at every level appreciate the review process. They accept it as being very positive and it is seen as being very much part of quality improvement and part of what we do. A number of the more significant incidents are reviewed and are reported at board level.

***

When I look back at my seven years as master, I do so with great pride. I have to thank the staff of the hospital, the management team and all of my consultant colleagues who supported me in the role. It really was a team effort. Together we managed the busiest time in the history of the hospital and maintained our performance outcomes despite the funding deficits and headcount restrictions. We managed to turn the reporting and committee structures around, so that responsibilities and accountabilities were much clearer, and we put clinical audit and research on a much better footing. We also advanced the idea of subspecialist services being made more available to other maternity units in the group. The appointment of some key personnel in the laboratories and in pharmacy, and joint appointments with the Mater raised the hospital's profile considerably. We managed the media well and the Rotunda became the go-to place when media outlets were looking for comment on important women's health issues. I learned a huge amount from women who had been affected by the organ retention issue, how their loss had stayed with them and how difficult it had been for them to deal with. As a result, we modified and improved our bereavement services to be a model for the country.

There were of course regrets and issues. The loss of our TCD undergraduate link was a blow, but our relationship with the RCSI has blossomed. Our inability to influence Professor Higgins and his strategy group on the establishment of hospital groups was also unfortunate. In my view it was a lost opportunity not to include the Mater in the North East Hospital Group, now the RCSI Hospital Group. We tried to convince Minister Mary Harney not to give the contract for our national cervical screening service to an American company, but sadly we failed and the consequences have been devastating for so many women and their families. There were several reports from external consultant groups looking at co-location and the site for the new children's hospital, and in my view a huge opportunity was missed. A tri-located Mater/Rotunda/children's hospital could have been delivered many years ago for a fraction of the cost of the new national children's hospital. Current government policy is to move us to Connolly. This is neither achievable nor sensible, and in my view should never happen.

In retrospect, with regard to the HSE, now that I have a better understanding of how that organisation works and am more aware of its attitude to voluntary hospitals, I am sorry we did not deal with this better. I think that both sides became too entrenched in their views and failed to understand each other.

If one were to ask former masters of any of the Irish maternity hospitals what their biggest challenge was, you can be guaranteed that their answer will include managing people, relationships and expectations. The key is communication and when communications are good, instructions are clear, messages are understood, expectations are defined and levels of frustration and complaint are reduced.

***

In 2010 during my mastership there was a really tragic maternal death of an African-born woman who died as a result of bleeding from a ruptured uterus. Her baby had died in utero and she was being induced because of this, which is normal practice. But what we did not know, and we do not think she knew either, because she did not volunteer it, was that at some time in her past she must have had a procedure which perforated the top of her uterus and this had left her with an inherent weakness in the wall of her uterus. When she started to contract, she ruptured her uterus and died as a result of bleeding. The case was examined by the Coroner's Court in 2013.

Events such as these are tragic and have a profound effect on everyone associated with them. We develop resilience because we have to, and I do not think it is possible to survive in obstetrics without it. From the earliest years of our careers, we are learning resilience – physical, mental and emotional. With each experience, we develop ways of dealing with situations, good and bad, and we watch how other people deal in similar circumstances. We listen to others, we share experiences and we realise that we are not on our own. The multiple knock-backs we experience and the way we and our colleagues around us handle them gives us the miles under our belts. Over time we build up a personal network of friends and colleagues who become our primary source of support. Offloading to colleagues at lunchtime or in the coffee room immediately after a bad situation is really important and helps considerably in how one deals with a poor outcome.

Obstetrics and gynaecology are areas of medicine where the doctors and midwives tend to have a great deal of empathy towards each other, as well as towards their patients. If you spend enough time in the labour ward and in theatre, you will come across difficult situations that are not necessarily anyone's fault. When something does go wrong, your heart does go out to everyone involved. It is a tragedy for both the patients and the family, as well as for the staff. There are many victims in these situations and it is very important from the Rotunda's management point of view that we ensure that in those stressful situations the staff as well as the patients are well looked after.

One of my concerns about the recent trend in appointing young consultants is that they have had shorter periods of intensive training but are being appointed to a high degree of responsibility without many years of experience. In my generation we were appointed as consultants in our forties after many years as senior registrars, but now consultants are being appointed in their thirties with perhaps only five years' experience as an SpR. Consequently, they have had less time on call, less exposure and less experience than we would have had. Each one of us has to find a way of dealing with stressful situations so as not to burn out. When someone is appointed as a consultant, they are thrown in at the deep end where they are expected to practise solo under pressure. When it comes to really difficult situations, it is clear that they may not be as comfortable dealing with those as we might have been, and it can be a lonely place when bad things inevitably happen. Some young consultants cope remarkably well, while others find it difficult.

Today the expectations of a good outcome are higher than they would have been in years gone by, and there is more pressure on the job even though the perinatal mortality rate in Dublin has dropped significantly over the last fifty years or so. In the past everyone knew someone who had had a baby who had died, or a pregnancy that did not have a good outcome or a cot death that had happened. Bad outcomes were not uncommon, but no one got sued. This is not the case today. Everyone expects to have a perfect baby when they become pregnant, and no one expects to miscarry. Women are putting off having babies until they are in their thirties, and then they are surprised when they have miscarriages. And forty-year-old mothers have babies with more abnormalities, which is just the way it is and is not anyone's fault. The pressure is on the younger consultants to deliver the perfect outcome, which can take its own toll.

***

Stepping back from the mastership in December 2015 was more difficult than I expected. Obviously, I knew it was coming, but it was still a bigger hit than I had anticipated. I returned to my former position as a consultant obstetrician in the hospital, which is an unusual arrangement. I cannot think of any other profession or business where the CEO of the organisation steps back to their former position in the same organisation. Managing that transition was difficult and I think it is a huge issue, not just for me but for other former masters of the Dublin maternity hospitals. In a conversation with Sean Daly, master of the Coombe from 1999 to 2005, he said to me that the hardest part of being master was no longer being master. That is actually very true.

One of the principal issues for the outgoing master is handling the loss of the sense of ownership and responsibility that has been with them for seven years. It is not unlike a bereavement and needs to be managed. When we commence our term of office, we have no idea what the reality is going to be at the end of it because it is a completely new experience. We have accepted a very intense role that makes enormous demands on us and when it is over, everything is stripped away very quickly. We know it is coming, it is inevitable, and we think we are ready, but when it happens it does not lessen the shock. We come to work every day still carrying that sense of ownership and responsibility but without having either anymore. I remember the first few days of January 2016, wondering where I should go when I arrived in the hospital each morning. It can be hard to watch decisions being made by the new master that we might not be in agreement with, or to see our policies being changed. I have discussed this matter with our Board of Governors and I believe they have a responsibility to the outgoing master to ensure that they are looked after appropriately. Each master gives of themselves massively during the course of those seven years and there is a duty of care that often may not be realised.

Besides the loss of the sense of responsibility at work, part of the impact of no longer being master is that when you come home, the family – partner and children – have moved on. They loaned you to the hospital for seven years and you expected them to have stayed still, waiting for you to return, but they have, of course, been doing their own thing and are busy getting on with their own lives. That takes some getting used to. You now have to catch up and adapt and roll with this new situation. And unless you are expecting it, it comes as a surprise. For me that was an important reflection. I became so wrapped up in my own world, and with the issues and concerns of the day-to-day running of the hospital, that it was easy to forget the other important aspects of life like family and relationships, all of which need just as much work and attention.

By the end of my mastership I realised how important it is that obstetricians and midwives draw on their own reserves and supports, professional and personal, because if we do not, we tend to layer up issues in the background and bury them. Over the course of my time as master, I had many different issues and concerns to deal with, as well as personal bereavements, including the deaths of my parents. I am sure I did not totally deal with all those things and in the two to three years after finishing the mastership I found myself being buried under all those layers. It was taking its toll until I found a skilled professional to help me to deal with all of that. There is a requirement on us all to look after each other and a personal requirement to ensure that we mind ourselves. If we do not, the unseen layers accumulate in the background and ultimately can catch up on us if we are not careful.

Some medical people develop a strategy in which they disassociate themselves from their work and its difficult outcomes. They have that ability. But I do not think it can be done completely. If one is going to learn from an experience, one has to take on board what has happened. There is a certain amount that you have to give into in order to learn, so it has to affect you at some level. If someone puts things behind them very quickly, it suggests that they have not analysed the situation appropriately and have not learned from it.

***

During the 2020–21 Covid pandemic, the health services have coped remarkably well, but it has taken its toll on people, and the staff of the Rotunda were no different, as everyone in the hospital found it tough. In a way we were lucky in that we were able to come to work and were not isolated at home, and we were lucky not to have too many sick patients. But as the months went on, the restrictions and social distancing wore people down and we had few social or physical outlets to deal with the strain. We could see that we were maybe a little bit more short-tempered, more easily stressed and perhaps not dealing with things quite as well because of that. We also recognised the stress and mental health issues for our patients, who were anxious and concerned about their own welfare and the welfare of their babies. The normal supports that pregnant women usually rely on – their partners, close families and friends – were not as easily accessible to them during social isolation. The patients were on their own for longer periods with only the staff to lean on, and this put an additional strain on the staff.

We did our best to maintain a degree of camaraderie among ourselves. We could meet for coffee in our coffee room wearing masks and with the windows open, or in the canteen for lunch, but with only two people at a table it was difficult. Our inability to unwind in the canteen, to offload and to share experiences started to show and our legendary collegiality was threatened.

Managing the stresses of the job is something we are getting better at recognising and dealing with. But there is still very much a culture in obstetrics that tough situations are part of the job and we just have to get on with it. That works for some people, but not for everybody. In the old days it was see one, do one, teach one and learn from your mistakes. That is not something that exists anymore, and we are much more aware of our trainees and we mind them much more carefully. This is something that is evolving as time goes on.

In 2019 I attended a doctors' update meeting at Val d'Isère in the French Alps with colleagues from the Rotunda. It is an annual multidisciplinary meeting for surgeons, physicians, anaesthetists, general practitioners and so on. It is an international gathering with a strong British base. There are updates on lots of different areas, which make it very interesting. And there is a lot of skiing involved, too, so it is a bit of fun. That year a number of presenters spoke about well-being at work. I had never really heard people talk about it before. The speakers were not talking about a particular piece of research but rather presenting it as an area that needs to be addressed and taken on board. I was absolutely astounded at the amount of information and knowledge that was brought into the discussions. It was a real eye-opener for me that people are developing an understanding about the impact of our kind of work on people's lives, and on the amount of alcohol, drug abuse and suicide that occurs in the medical profession. This is a much bigger deal than I had actually realised. I knew it happened but did not realise that it happened to the extent that was being presented to us. There are now people whose job is to examine this area and to find ways of improving the work–life balance and managing stress for health care workers. It is something that we need to be much better at for ourselves and for our staff, and something we need to address in a practical way, especially following the Covid pandemic. It is likely that a voluntary hospital would have to take a lead on this before it is rolled out across the hospital network in Ireland.

14

CONCLUSION
VOLUNTARY HOSPITALS:
DELIVERING THE FUTURE

• • • • • • • • •

The Irish voluntary hospitals that have survived to 2021 have retained the characteristics that make them more efficient, more strategic and more innovative than most state hospitals. But where do we go from here? On the one hand the voluntary hospitals, including the Rotunda, provide leadership to the Irish health system and house all the national specialties. We are centres for innovation and quality improvement, and we create an environment for our staff to flourish. We attract great staff, undertake research, think strategically, are accountable and responsible, and focus on clinical outcomes for patients. As the hospital group system evolves, subspecialist clinical staff based in the major teaching hospitals are providing services to regional hospitals on a part-time basis through the hub-and-spoke model.

On the other hand, our independence is being steadily eroded through government policies that do not recognise or perhaps even understand the value of the voluntary hospitals. The hospital groups were put in place in 2013 without the necessary thought about how they were going to function properly with voluntary hospitals involved with them. The groups other than the Children's Hospital Group did not – and still do not – have any statutory power and therefore do not exist as legal entities, while the voluntary hospitals have their own legal, independent status. Each year we are obliged to sign SLAs that contain clauses that further compromise and erode our independence. And while this bureaucracy imposes controls and restrictions on us, when we have a major crisis in the hospital, we are told that it is our risk and we have to manage it ourselves. We have all the responsibility and accountability, but the power and the funds to solve major problems lie with the government authorities. A middle ground is the way forward, a place where relationships can flourish, where mutual respect is the norm and where working partnerships exist.

It was a relief to many of us working in the voluntary sector that the report of the IRG led by Catherine Day recognised the value of the voluntary sector and acknowledged the frustrations and difficulties we face in our dealings with the state health authorities. The IRG report went as far as to say that the relationship between the Irish health services and the voluntary sector was fractured. The IRG's research into the positive ways in which other countries blend voluntary and public hospitals was included briefly in the report and showed that it is possible to build a service around the different styles of hospital to create an integrated service.

***

Each year we talk about a health budget that is being blown out of the water and in the midst of a pandemic it is an awkward question to ask, but is the administration of the health service costing significantly more than it ever did before? The Irish health authorities have a wide remit, managing community services, hospital services, general practice and so on. With the hospital groups, they have divested some of their administrative function, but have they downsized themselves in order to do that? There are huge numbers of people working within the Irish health service whose job is to manage budgets, manage people and process information.

In an ideal world there would be a health service where the state authorities provide national direction for the hospital sector, look after the national procurement of supplies, and provide the necessary environment and equipment for us to do what we need to do. Then, in this ideal world, they would trust the hospitals to manage the day-to-day activities and to develop necessary services based on information from clinical data. The voluntary hospitals do not need to be controlled or micromanaged. We have governance structures that keep a very close eye on what is happening in our institutions. Our boards are obliged to comply with national legislation as well as guidelines, standards, regulations and other frameworks, and to make sure that the hospitals remain financially viable. In addition, as charitable organisations, we are mandated by law to manage our finances. Therefore, once the boards are doing their job, the hospitals do not need the extra layer of policing by the state health authorities that takes so much time and effort on both parts. Occasionally there are voluntary institutions that do not play by the rules, but these are the exception and are not a reason for the health authorities to distrust all of the hospitals' financial management and compliance.

The Covid pandemic has shown how voluntary hospitals within the health service can be an incredibly valuable asset and can adapt, respond and act in a way that the state hospitals cannot. We have shown that if you give clinicians the freedom to use their skills and abilities, they will respond appropriately. The IRG report identified this characteristic of the voluntary organisations: 'there is more autonomy and authority at local management level [in the voluntary organisations] which encourages a more prompt, flexible and responsive approach to problem-solving and supports the piloting of quality improvement initiatives.'[1] The HSE acknowledged the voluntary sector's contribution in their 2020 annual report:

> In responding to COVID-19, we relied heavily on the expertise of the voluntary health sector (section 38 and 39 agencies) to deliver a substantial element of health and social care services. The work undertaken underscores the importance of continuing to build on these relationships, grounded on mutual trust and respect, recognising and working collaboratively to address the particular challenges faced by our voluntary partners.[2]

If we want to maintain that sort of quality, leadership and adaptability, then the voluntary hospitals have to be recognised in law as a group within our health services.

I know that the state health authorities find this difficult because it is used to controlling its own hospitals. However, I would further suggest that the controls over all public hospitals should be loosened and their staff trusted to deliver the best services, because at the moment most state hospitals do not have that freedom. There is very little service development in most regional state hospitals. They provide a service and that is where it begins and ends. Their management cannot think ahead in terms of where they want to be or what they want to do because there are so many hoops that these hospitals need to jump through, meaning their ability to adapt is just far too slow. However, if their hospitals were to be turned into voluntary-style hospitals with a board to oversee the service close to home, there would be better quality outcomes and better quality services and probably better financial management because there would be local accountability.

In order to carry the benefits of the voluntary hospitals' management style into the future, the relationship between the voluntary hospitals and the state authorities has to be resolved. It is not a healthy working relationship and the IRG report identified many frustrating issues, especially around budgets and SLAs. Each year conditions in the SLAs undermine our autonomy a little bit more. If we do not sign them, we are threatened with a percentage of our budget being withheld, so many of the hospitals sign them with extensive exclusion clauses. This approach, as the IRG report pointed out, is burdensome and 'could not be accurately described as a "negotiation" at all'.[3]

In 2021, eight years after they were created, the lack of thought concerning governance of the hospital groups is yet to be resolved. If, as in the RCSI Group, the major voluntary hospital in each group provides some services to regional hospitals in a hub-and-spoke model, the question arises as to where the governance for those services lies. Is the governance under a state health organisation or under the voluntary hospital that is providing the services? It is questionable whether the legal status of the voluntary hospitals is truly understood by the state health authorities, including the Department of Health, because, in developing the service arrangement, the authorities do so without a recognition or understanding of the role of the governance structure of the voluntary hospitals. The SLA becomes the de facto governance model for the state for the voluntary sector and without good understanding between the state authorities and the voluntary hospitals, the SLA actually deepens the severing of the relationship and the lack of understanding between the two parties.

It is possible that the findings of the IRG report, together with the voluntary organisations' response to the Covid pandemic may be the start of a new relationship of mutual respect and appreciation for our respective roles. We would like much more of a partnership with the groups and the state health authorities in terms of managing risk and delivering quality healthcare. In a conversation with me, Paul Reid, director-general of the HSE, said:

> I never knew the distinction between some of the section 38s [voluntary hospitals] and others. I just knew that they were part of the system, and I know that some of the board structures, some of the governance structures were slightly different but I just viewed them as part of the system ... I do think the partnership approach you talk about is definitely something we could work on.

To move this forward, the conversation with the state health care authorities and the voluntary hospitals needs to be less about the budget and monitoring compliance, and more about clinical care and development.

When mutual trust is established, the voluntary hospitals can contribute actively to the improvement and development of the Irish hospital system. We can use our wisdom and experience to support the state authorities in the development of overarching policy and strategic development. We can share expertise, develop services, make cross-appointments and provide information to regional hospitals in the group. In return we would appreciate input from the state health authorities when it comes to helping us solve some of the major issues we face in delivering our services. In a new atmosphere of trust, it would be hoped that the head of a voluntary hospital is never again told that a major crisis is their risk and they have to manage it.

In a recent podcast by David McWilliams, he explored how women's leadership styles have had an impact, and wondered if a bank run by 'Lehmann Sisters' rather than the Lehmann Brothers would have taken such risks and contributed to the collapse of economies in 2008. Prompted by this podcast, I wondered whether a woman would have dismissed me by telling me it was my risk when I presented the difficult and potentially dangerous situation a major maternity hospital was facing. There have always been women serving at board level in the Rotunda, whether that was organising charity for our patients or, in more recent years, serving on the Board of Governors. Gordon Linney pointed out that women have brought a softness to the management of the hospital.[4] There are numerous women in senior positions in the state health authorities and I can only speculate on whether one of them may have been more empathetic to the conditions our patients were facing when I was seeking practical support.

***

In conclusion the situation, as it is now, is that if no one rocks the boat too much, we will just evolve into something that is slightly different from what we have now. The trouble is no one knows or has a plan about what that is. If the attitude towards the voluntary hospitals is changing at the top and state health-care authorities accept that the voluntary hospitals are good at minding money and staying within all regulations, it is time to find a way to trust us to get on with it. I am asking for the recognition that this is a complex situation and that ideally someone somewhere needs to be put in charge of the next stage in the evolution of the health service. Much of what I am saying is backed up by the IRG report. There is a lot of valuable and high-quality work happening in the voluntary hospitals, so let us accept that these are mostly good, well-run institutions that are used to managing a budget and are good at what they do, and trust them. If the voluntary hospitals are brought down to the level of state hospitals, then the country is going to lose the agility, flexibility and expertise that is required for service development, let alone crisis management. And if something is not done to address this, the influence of the state health authorities, including the groups, will grow and eventually take over, and our health service will be the poorer because of it.

My concern and my motivation in writing this book is to get the message about the true value of the voluntary hospitals across to the next generation of doctors, midwives, nurses and other medical staff, and to politicians, civil servants and the general public, because in fifteen or twenty years' time we are at risk that people will not understand what voluntarism means and why it is so important. It is up to us in the voluntary sector to fight our corner and let it be heard that the country needs voluntary hospitals. Without them, our ability to respond to change, to adapt and to provide medical leadership will be lost. We need a vibrant voluntary sector to deliver health care in the country, now and into the future. The place of voluntary hospitals needs to be protected by legislation so it is enshrined, nourished and protected. My hope for this book is that I have demonstrated how, especially over the last twenty to thirty years, voluntary hospitals have provided that leadership and have responded to the needs of patients as individuals and the country as a whole when it comes to times of difficulty. As a country we would be poorer without this sector, and our contribution to how the Covid crisis was managed was a very good example of that. I hope that those in charge recognise this and are able to maintain a trusted and partnership approach rather than a controlling one.

APPENDIX:
MASTERS OF THE
ROTUNDA HOSPITAL

1745–1759	Bartholomew Mosse
1759–1766	Fielding Ould
1766–1773	William Collum
1773–1780	Frederick Jebb
1780–1786	Henry Rock
1786–1793	Joseph Clarke
1793–1800	Thomas Evory
1800–1807	Thomas Kelly
1807–1814	Francis Hopkins
1814–1821	Samuel Labatt
1821–1826	John Pentland
1826–1833	Robert Collins
1833–1840	Evory Kennedy
1840–1847	Charles Johnson
1847–1854	Robert Shekleton
1854–1861	Alfred McClintock
1861–1868	John Denham

1868–1875	George Johnston
1875–1882	Lombe Atthill
1882–1889	Arthur Vernon Macan
1889–1896	William Smyly
1896–1903	Richard Dancer Purefoy
1903–1910	Ernest Tweedy
1910–1919	Henry Jellett
1919–1926	Gibbon Fitzgibbon
1926–1933	Bethel Solomons
1933–1940	Andrew Davidson
1940–1947	Ninian McIntire Falkiner
1947–1952	O'Donel Thornley Dodwell Browne
1952–1959	Eric Thompson
1960–1966	Alan Browne
1967–1973	Edwin Lillie
1974–1980	Ian Dalrymple
1981–1987	George Henry
1988–1994	Michael Darling
1995–2001	Peter McKenna
2002–2008	Mike Geary
2009–2015	Sam Coulter-Smith
2016–present	Fergal Malone

ENDNOTES

Foreword

1 Department of Health, *Report of the Independent Review Group established to examine the Role of Voluntary Organisations in Public Health and Personal Social Care Settings* (hereafter IRG report) (February 2019), p. 60.
2 Ibid.
3 *National Economic & Social Council, Building a New Relationship between Voluntary Organisations and the State in the Health and Social Care Sectors* (July 2021).

Introduction

1 IRG report, op. cit., p. 11.
2 *HSE Annual Report and Financial Statements 2019*, https://www.hse. ie/eng/services/publications/corporate/hse-annual-report-and-financial-statements-2019.pdf, p. 24.
3 IRG report, op. cit., pp. 5–6.
4 Ibid., p. 33.
5 Ibid.
6 Ibid., p. 60.
7 Ibid., p. 57.
8 Author in conversation with Paul Reid, March 2021.
9 Ibid.
10 IRG report, op. cit., p. 6.
11 Ibid., p. 11.

1. The Journey So Far

1 Browne, O'Donel, *The Rotunda Hospital 1745–1945* (Edinburgh: E&S Livingstone, 1947), p. 17.

2 Henry Rock and John Pentland died in office in 1786 and 1826 respectively; and while Henry Jellett served on the continent, three former masters, Smyly, Purefoy and Tweedy acted in the role from 1915–17.

3 Browne, O'Donel, op. cit., p. 18.

4 Ibid., pp. 47–9.

5 O Gráda, Cormac, 'The Rotunda and the people of Dublin 1745–1995' in Alan Browne (ed.), *Masters, Midwives and Ladies-in-waiting: the Rotunda Hospital 1745–1995* (Dublin: A.&A. Farmar, 1995), pp. 247–8.

6 Holmes, in Browne, Alan, op. cit., pp. 230–1.6 Whitfield, Ann, 'A short history of Obstetric Anaesthesia', *Res Medica: Journal of the Royal Medical Society*, Vol. 3, No. 1 (1992), pp. 28–30.

7 Browne, O'Donel, op. cit., p. 276.

8 Kirkpatrick, T. Percy C., *The Book of the Rotunda Hospital: An Illustrated History of the Dublin Lying-In Hospital from its Foundation in 1745 to the Present Time,* edited by Henry Jellett (London, Adlard & Son, Bartholomew Press, 1913), pp. 184–5.

9 Browne, O'Donel, op. cit., p. 52; beds, p. 58; swing cots, p. 71.

10 https://theconversation.com/ignaz-semmelweis-the-doctor-who-dis covered-the-disease-fighting-power-of-hand-washing-in-1847-135528.

11 Keenan, Desmond, *Post-famine Ireland: Social Structure* (second ed., Xlibris, 2019), p. 740.

12 Kirkpatrick and Jellett, op. cit., p. 183.

13 Browne, O'Donel, op. cit., p. 275.

14 Robins, Joseph, 'Public policy and the maternity services in Ireland during the twentieth century', in Alan Browne, op. cit., pp. 292.

15 Kirkpatrick and Jellett, op. cit., pp. 179–80.

16 Kelly, Mary A., 'The development of midwifery at the Rotunda', in Alan Browne, op. cit., p. 101.

17 Midwives (Ireland) Act 1918. Act controlling unqualified persons from practising midwifery was tightened up by the Midwives Act, 1931, and Midwives Act 1944.

18 Holmes, Eleanor A., 'Medical social work at the Rotunda', in Alan Browne, op. cit., p. 210.

19 Robins, in Browne, Alan, op. cit., p. 292.

20 KPMG, *Independent Review of Maternity and Gynaecology Services in the Greater Dublin Area* (2008), p. 185.

21 Browne, O'Donel, op. cit., pp. 81–2.

22 KPMG report, op. cit., p. 21.

2. Centre of Excellence

1 Steven Brody, 'The Life and Times of Sir Fielding Ould: Man-Midwife and Master Physician', *Bulletin of Medicine*, Vol. 52, No. 2 (Summer 1978), pp. 228–50, see p. 228.

2 Harrison, Robert F., 'Medical education at the Rotunda Hospital 1745–1995', in Alan Browne, op. cit., p. 71.

3 Ibid., p. 68.

4 Browne, O'Donel, op. cit., p. 41.

5 Kelly, in Browne, Alan, op. cit., p. 79.

6 Harrison, in Browne, Alan, op. cit., p. 67; in 1848 Corson from the USA said no practice was better than that in the Rotunda; in 1851 Arneth said it was the only one of importance in Britain and Ireland. In the 1950s the General Medical Council and American Medical Association commented favourably on the quality of instruction in the Rotunda.

7 Kirkpatrick and Jellett, op. cit., pp. 187–8.

8 Kelly, in Browne, Alan, op. cit., p. 95.

9 Ibid., p. 105.

10 Browne, O'Donel, op. cit., p. 272.

11 Harrison, in Browne, Alan, op. cit., pp. 69–70.

12 Gardiner, James, 'Clinical specialities' in Alan Browne, op. cit., p. 184.

3. In Pursuit of Quality

1 Browne, O'Donel, op. cit., p. 262.

2 Kirkpatrick and Jellett, op. cit., p. 150.

3 Ibid., p. 155.

4 Walsh, Oonagh, *Report on Symphysiotomy in Ireland, 1944–1984* (Department of Health, 2014), p. 31.

5 Ibid., p. 4.

6 Clark, Maureen Harding, *The Lourdes Hospital Inquiry: An Inquiry into Peripartum Hysterectomy at Our Lady of Lourdes Hospital, Drogheda* (Department of Health and Children, 2006), pp. 39 and 135.

7 Ibid., p. 164.

8 Ibid., pp. 169–70.

9 Ibid., pp. 83–4. No figures were given for the Rotunda.

10 *Creating a Better Future Together: National Maternity Strategy 2016–2026*, pp. 73–6.

11 https://www.hse.ie/eng/about/who/acute-hospitals-division/woman-infants/.

12 Royal College of Physicians of Ireland, *The National Clinical Programme for Obstetrics and Gynaecology, HSE and Institute of Obstetricians and Gynaecologists* (RCPI, 2015).

13 The author in conversation with Mike Turner, March 2021.

4. Pushing the Boundaries

1 Browne, 'Mastership in action at the Rotunda 1945–95', in Alan Browne, op. cit., p. 41.

2 Kirkpatrick and Jellett, pp. 106ff.

3 Browne, O'Donel, op. cit., pp. 122–3.

4 In 1934 Solomons was awarded the Honorary Fellowship of the American College of Surgeons and was made an Honorary Fellow of the American Association of Obstetricians, Gynaecologists and Abdominal Surgeons, an Honorary Member of the Central Association of Obstetricians of

America and a member of the Association d'Enseignement Médical Complementaire. Browne, O'Donel, op. cit., pp. 81–2.

5   Browne, 'Mastership in action at the Rotunda 1945–95', in Alan Browne, op. cit., pp. 28–9.

6   Ibid., p. 41.

7   Ibid.

8   Email from Brian Cleary to the author, 29 June 2021.

9   The Abortion Act 1967, Britain legalised abortion up to twenty-eight weeks' gestation; reduced to twenty-four weeks in 1990.

10 Traditionally the MRCOG is the postgraduate exam that carries most weight in Ireland in terms of an obstetrics and gynaecology qualification and in terms of progressing a career. Many students will also do the obstetric version of the MRCPI.

5. Obstetrics in Dublin: A Historical Perspective

1   Walsh, op. cit., p. 29.

2   Barrington, Ruth, *Health, Medicine & Politics in Ireland 1900–1970* (Dublin: Institute of Public Administration 1987), pp. 14–15.

3   Fleetwood, John F., *The History of Medicine in Ireland* (The Skellig Press, 1983), pp. 123–4.

4   Browne, O'Donel, op. cit., pp. 60–1.

5   IRG report, op. cit., pp. 76–83.

6   Walsh, op. cit., p. 19.

7   Solomons, Michael, *Pro Life? The Irish Question* (Dublin: The Lilliput Press, 1992), p. 5.

8   Fleetwood, op. cit., p. 121.

9   Browne, O'Donel, op. cit., p. 206.

10 Ibid., p. 225.

11 Walsh, op. cit., p. 18.

12 Solomons, op. cit., pp. 5–7.

13 Ibid., p. 14.

14 Ibid., p. 6

15 Browne, O'Donel, op. cit., p. 172.

16 Ibid., p. 184.

17 Walsh, op. cit., p. 18.

18 Ibid., pp. 22–3.

19 Ibid., pp. 8–9.

20 Quote from Jacqueline Morrissey, in *The Irish Times*, 6 September 1999. Walsh, op. cit., p. 30.

21 *Western Journal of Medicine* 2000 Apr; 172(4): 240–243; sourced 21/10/2020.https://www.ncbi.nlm.nih.gov/pmc/articles/PMC1070831/#:~:text=The%20active%20management%20of%20labor,short%20labors%20in%20nulliparous%20women.

22 Boylan, Peter, *In the Shadow of the Eighth: Forty Years Working for Women's Health in Ireland* (London: Penguin, 2020), pp. 14–15.

6. Promoting Innovation

1 Mellow in Browne, Alan, op. cit., pp. 164–7; see also Horst Dickel 'Hans Sachs' in *German-speaking Exiles in Ireland 1933–1945*, available at https://brill.com/view/book/edcoll/9789401203227/B9789401203227-s012.xml.

2 https://en.wikipedia.org/wiki/Hans_Sachs_(serologist), accessed 10 February 2021.

3 Browne, O'Donel, op. cit., p. 94.

4 Holmes, in Browne, Alan, op. cit., p. 200.

5 Ibid., p. 216.

6 Clark, op. cit., pp. 169–70.

7 IRG report, op. cit., p. 72.

8 Ibid., p. 34.

9 Ibid., p. 67.

7. Leadership in Practice

1 KPMG, op. cit., p. 21.

2 Kirkpatrick and Jellett, op. cit., p. 159.

3 Mosse lived in the hospital. When Frederick Jebb was appointed in 1774, the governors decided that master was to reside in the hospital with his family. It was strictly observed. Kirkpatrick and Jellett, op. cit., p. 85.

4 Kirkpatrick and Jellett, op. cit., pp. 159–60.

5 IRG report, op. cit., p. 33.

6 Ibid., p. 44.

7 Author in conversation with Reverend Gordon Linney, March 2021.

8 Kelly, in Browne, Alan, op. cit., p. 100.

9 Browne, O'Donel, op. cit., pp. 79–80.

10 Ibid., pp. 79–81.

11 Solomons, op. cit., p. 34.

12 Darling, Michael, 'Michael R.N. Darling, master 1988–94', in Alan Browne, op. cit., p. 57.

13 Angela Fitzgerald in conversation with the author.

14 Clark, op. cit., p. 170.

15 Ibid., p. 158.

16 Michael Turner in conversation with the author, 2021.

17 KPMG, op. cit., p. 21.

18 Ibid.

8. Health Care and the State

1 *Outline of the Future Hospital System Report of the Consultative Council on General Hospital Services* [Fitzgerald report] (Dublin, 1968).

2 Robins, in Browne, Alan, op. cit., pp. 295–6.

3 IRG report, op. cit., p. 24.

4 Kirkpatrick and Jellett, op. cit., p. 133.

5 Browne, O'Donel, op. cit., p. 282.

6 O Gráda, in Browne, Alan, op. cit., p. 245.

7 Browne, O'Donel, op. cit., p. 82; Robins, in Browne, Alan, op. cit., p. 287.

8 Kelly, in Browne, Alan, op. cit., p. 96.

9 IRG report, op. cit., p. 39.

9. The Mastership: Learning to Manage Risk

1   Holmes, in Browne, Alan, op. cit., pp. 230–1.

2   The Rotunda Hospital, *Corporate Report 2014* (Dublin, 2014), p. 29.

10. The Mastership: Expecting the Unexpected

1   *The Irish Times*, 29 January 2017 and 11 February 2017.

2   IRG report, op. cit., p. 63.

3   Ibid.

4   Ibid.

5   Ibid., pp. 11–12.

6   Brian Cleary in an email to the author, 2021.

7   Arulkumaran, Sabaratnam, *Investigation of Incident 50278 from time of patient's self-referral to hospital on the 21st of October 2012 to the patient's death on the 28th of October, 2012* (HSE, 2013).

8   Ibid., p. 13.

9   Ibid., p. 17.

11. Shifting Sands: Government Policy and the Hospitals

1   Directors of the TUH, https://www.tuh.ie/About-us/Hospital-Board.html, accessed 17 February.

2   Author in conversation with Reverend Gordon Linney, February 2021.

3   Higgins, John R., Chair of the Strategic Board, *The Establishment of Hospital Groups as a Transition to Independent Hospital Trusts: A report to the Minister for Health, Dr James Reilly, TD* (Department of Health, 2013), pp. 63–4.

4   Wall, Martin, 'Rotunda's move to Connolly cold take up to 10 years', *The Irish Times,* 14 August 2018.

5   Author in conversation with Peter McKenna, February 2021.

6   The other regional areas are Area B: Dublin west, Westmeath, Kildare, Offaly, Laois and Longford; Area C: Wicklow, Kilkenny, Carlow, Tipperary South, Waterford and Wexford; Area D: Cork and Kerry; Area

E: Limerick, Tipperary north and Clare; Area F: Galway, Mayo, Leitrim, Roscommon, Sligo and Donegal.

7 Walls, Martin, 'Health and social care to be delivered through six new regions', *The Irish Times*, 17 July 2019.

8 Boylan, op. cit.

12. The Latest Developments

1 Author in conversation with Mike Turner, March 2021.

2 Author in conversation with Peter McKenna, February 2021.

3 The OECD (Organisation for Economic Co-operation and Development) is an intergovernmental economic organisation with thirty-eight member countries, including Ireland.

4 Author in conversation with Mike Turner, March 2021.

5 IRG report, op. cit., p. 11.

6 *Voluntary Organisations Dialogue Forum Terms of Reference* (Department of Health, 2020), p. 1.

7 *Building a New Relationship between Voluntary Organisations and the State in the Health and Social Care Sectors* (National Economic and Social Council, 2021), p. 2.

8 Ibid.

14. Conclusion: Voluntary Hospitals: Delivering the Future

1 IRG report, op. cit., p. 33.

2 Health Service Executive, op. cit., p. 23.

3 IRG report, op. cit., p. 63.

4 Author in conversation with Reverend Gordon Linney, February 2021.

SELECT BIBLIOGRAPHY

Barrington, Ruth, *Health, Medicine & Politics in Ireland 1900–1970* (Dublin: Institute of Public Administration, 1987).

Browne, Alan (ed.), *Masters, Midwives and Ladies-in-Waiting: The Rotunda Hospital 1745–1995* (Dublin: A.&A. Farmar, 1995).

Browne, O'Donel, *The Rotunda Hospital 1745–1945* (Edinburgh: E&S Livingstone, 1947).

Clark, Maureen Harding, *The Lourdes Hospital Inquiry: An Inquiry into Peripartum Hysterectomy at Our Lady of Lourdes Hospital, Drogheda* (Department of Health & Children, 2006).

Department of Health, *The Establishment of Hospital Groups as a Transition to Independent Hospital Trusts A report to the Minister for Health, Dr James Reilly TD* (2013).

Department of Health, *Creating A Better Future Together: National Maternity Strategy, 2016–2026* (2016).

Department of Health, *Report of the Independent Review Group Established to Examine the Role of Voluntary Organisations in Publicly-Funded Health and Personal Social Services* (February 2019).

Health Service Executive, *Health Service Executive Annual Report and Financial Statements* (HSE, 2021)

Fleetwood, John F., *The History of Medicine in Ireland* (Dublin: The Skellig Press, 1983).

Kirkpatrick, T. Percy C., *The Book of the Rotunda Hospital: An Illustrated History of the Dublin Lying-In Hospital from its Foundation in 1745 to the Present Time*, edited by Henry Jellett (London: Adlard & Son, Bartholomew Press, 1913).

KPMG, *Independent Review of Maternity and Gynaecology Services in the Greater Dublin Area* (Dublin: HSE, 2008).

Solomons, Michael, *Pro Life? The Irish Question* (Dublin: The Lilliput Press, 1992).

Walsh, Oonagh, *Report on Symphysiotomy in Ireland, 1944–1984* (Department of Health, 2014).

ACKNOWLEDGEMENTS

As someone who has never written a book before, I really did not know where to start and this project would never have been completed without help and support from so many people.

It is not often that one gets an opportunity to formally and publicly thank one's loved ones, so firstly I want to acknowledge and thank Cathy, my wife, and my children, Sam, Katie and Lucy, for encouraging me to take on the role of master and supporting me in that job, for loaning me out for seven years, and for taking me back afterwards and putting up with what they got back until I sorted myself out.

I had a team of helpers who contributed to putting the book together: Catherine de Courcy, who assisted me with the multiple drafts of the manuscript. Her unerring eye for detail and probing questions got me on the right track, and her patience and determination I tested to the limit during the whole process. She deserves great credit and I cannot thank her enough. Those who agreed to be interviewed and contributed to the text were: Catherine Day, Gordon Linney, Hilary Prentice, Peter McKenna, Mike Turner, Bill Blunnie, Patricia Doherty, Paul Reid and Peter Boylan. Those who were my trusted readers and advisors: Liz McKeever, Anne O'Byrne, Cathy Madigan, Cedric Christie, Anne Brady, John Gleeson and Terry Prone. Sincere thanks to Ruth Barrington for writing the foreword; there are few people in Ireland who understand the evolution of our health system better.

ACKNOWLEDGEMENTS

Irish Academic Press who, having seen two chapters in draft, decided to take a flyer on the text.

To one and all, my thanks and gratitude.

INDEX